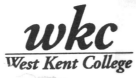

wkc
West Kent College

What Mak before the date last
You Tick?
is granted

What Makes You Tick?

THE BRAIN IN PLAIN ENGLISH

Thomas B. Czerner, M.D.

John Wiley & Sons, Inc.

Published by John Wiley & Sons, Inc., New York
Published simultaneously in Canada

This publication is designed to provide accurate and authoritative
information in regard to the subject matter covered. It is sold with
the understanding that the publisher is not engaged in rendering
professional services. If professional advice or other expert
assistance is required, the services of a competent professional
person should be sought.

Library of Congress Cataloging-in-Publication Data:

Czerner, Thomas B.
    What makes you tick? : the brain in plain English / Thomas B. Czerner.
        p. cm.
    Includes bibliographical references and index.
    ISBN 0-471-37100-9 (cloth : alk. paper)
    ISBN 0-471-20990-2 (paper)
    1. Brain. 2. Neurosciences. 3. Neuropsychology. I. Title.

OP376.C97 2000
612.8'2—dc21

                                        00-026289

For Cynthia,
who makes me tick

Contents

Preface
xi

Introduction
1

1
Exploring a Recently Discovered Galaxy
Off to See the Wizard
7

2
Stardust and the Music of the Neuron
Impulses and How They Move You
42

3
The Ghost in the Machine
The Elusive Homunculus
66

CONTENTS

4

The Photon and Your Brain
Your Quiet Conversation with Nature
76

5

The Intelligence of the Neuron
Your Life Depends on the Decisions of Individual Cells
89

6

The Moving Parts of Your Brain
*The Photon Illuminates the Lilliputian Machinery
of the Neuron*
101

7

The Yellow Brick Road
*To Your Biological Clock and Internal Maps
of the Universe*
120

8

The Emerald City
*The Secrets of the Most Complex Functions
of the Brain*
129

CONTENTS

9

Beyond the Yellow Brick Road
The Brain Is a Supercomputer and Much, Much More
148

10

The Shape of an Idea
Neuronal Ensembles
166

11

Pure Wizardry
Matching Your Behavior to Your Situation
180

12

Your Personal Chemistry
From Molecules to Moods and from Genes to Behavior
188

13

The Final Chord
207

Notes
213

Index
221

Preface

THIS BOOK OWES its beginnings to Dr. Erwin Froehlich, who knew me in Prague when I was too young to hold on to my memory of him. I came to know my maternal uncle from his powerful presence in tiny photographs. While growing up in Chicago, I would often pry them free of the small, black triangles that held their corners to a heavy album and bring them to the light. In fading shades of brown and gray, they framed his white coat and stethoscope and held his bright, kind, spectacled face. This was a face a nephew could love, trying without success to conceal his buoyant youth behind a serious, professional demeanor.

I was told about his academic accomplishments, his published clinical research, the free clinics he conducted, and how he loved to play with my two sisters and me. But I learned the truly important things about him, the things that mark a hero to a young boy, during the short pauses in those narratives, in the fleeting glimpse of a reflective smile on an older face filled with love and respect. I sensed the earnest warmth he radiated during those deceitfully promising years, the years before his unwilling ashes added to the darkness that hung over

Auschwitz, and over all of us.* I have often felt his gentle hand help to shape my life and work.

Similar images resonate in far too many family albums. Like shocking, miniature renditions of Picasso's painting *The Bombing of Guernica,* their impact reminds us that inhumanity is all too human. They implore us to discover what distinguishes the mind of a Mengele from that of a Mozart, to learn the critical differences between a Timothy McVeigh and a Mother Teresa, to explore the brain and to learn what special conditions must be met to cause human behavior and humane behavior to be one and the same. The good news is, we have begun.

---

*Despite frenzied efforts to legally emigrate anywhere in the world, Erwin and his mother, my grandmother Paula Froehlich, were trapped in that unspeakable scheme and met brutal ends alone—she at Treblinka and he at Auschwitz.

Introduction

THE ORGAN THAT GOVERNS your life has all of the elegance of a wrinkled lump of clay. It appears to have no moving parts and yet, if you damage one area, you cannot see, another and you cannot speak, another and you cannot walk. A source of speculation and mystery since its anatomy was first described in 300 B.C., the brain is giving up its secrets—only guessed at for centuries—to a young and ambitious branch of science. Ours is the first generation able to credibly answer the question *What makes you tick?* We are learning the lyrics of molecular melodies that create your perceptions and are deciphering the electrochemical signals that direct your behavior from the dark confines of your cranium. Simply put, we are beginning to fathom the biomechanics of human nature. The neurophilosopher Paul Churchland did not exaggerate when he wrote that today's revolutionary advances in neuroscience will rival the discoveries of Copernicus, Galileo, and Darwin.[1]

You are about to enter the most astonishing galaxy in the universe. Fueled by a mixture of science, technology, and philosophy, this expedition through the brain's billions of neurons will follow the paths of explorers from fields as diverse as molecular biology, computer science, evolutionary psychology, and a long list of disciplines, most of whose names begin with the prefix *neuro,* as in neuroanatomy, -audiology, -chemistry, -ophthalmology, -philosophy, -physiology, -radiology, and more.

With so many possible approaches, it should not surprise you that, as an ophthalmologist, I would choose the perception of light as a particularly revealing place to begin.

The eye has been called the window to the soul, and from the start the mystifying phenomenon of vision has been at the very heart of neuroscience. Soon after I finished medical school in the 1960s, a small band of researchers set out in earnest to learn the elusive secrets of the brain. Among their new set of tools were microelectrodes capable of recording the faint signals of an individual nerve cell. Like tapped phone conversations in a strange land, recordings of the neural signals from the eyes have taught us the language of the brain and, as our recording devices improve, they are disclosing the remarkable individuality, even intelligence of the single neuron.

The demarcating decade of the 1960s treated us to breathtaking views of our beautiful, blue planet from the sobering vantage point of space. It permanently imprinted us with surreal images of men loping oddly on the surface of the moon. At the same time, with little public fanfare, the race into outer space sparked an explosion of research into the equally mysterious inner reaches of the brain. The same advances in microengineering and computer technology that made space travel possible also provided the hardware, software, and the tiny tools necessary for entering inner space. As our horizon expanded to encompass light-years, we also learned to navigate on a scale measured in millionths of a millimeter. An exploration was launched at prestigious universities around the world in search of nothing less elusive than the source of human thought and behavior.

Nearly everything we know about the constellations of neurons in the brain we have learned in the past few decades, most of that only within the last few years, and the pace is picking up briskly. Brain mapping is being carried out at microscopic

2

levels. The structure of human DNA is available on the Internet. Direct links are being discovered between particular molecules and specific behavior. Researchers in more than a dozen disciplines are asking Plato's question: How does your internal representation of the world relate to the objective world outside? How does the electrochemical music of the neuron form perceptions, memories, and knowledge? How does it create the mystifying, subjective sense of a "you" within you, and how does it direct your individual and social behavior? Science has joined philosophy in this accelerating effort to define what it means to be alive, and to find the wellspring of our humanity.

No longer guessing the location of continents, today's explorers are probing the minute fissures, cells, and molecules that shape every aspect of your lively encounter with the world. The fanciful, intuitive maps of the human brain, which have guided this search in the past, are rapidly being replaced by precise navigational charts of the most complex three pounds of matter ever encountered.

Sadly, reports of this research are relished almost exclusively by a small community of neuroscientists. Even in the journals where they appear, the best parts are often hidden in the equations and technical jargon that have become a separate language of the laboratory. This book began as a personal, Berlitz guide for exploring that foreign territory, and it grew from a desire to make this adventure accessible to every curious traveler.

It is difficult to overstate the practical implications of this new wealth of knowledge. Understanding brain function at the level of detail now being studied holds the promise to cure and prevent a long list of diseases including Alzheimer's, schizophrenia, and drug addiction; to repair damaged nervous tissue; and to reverse the debility dealt by stroke and injury. Neuroscience will revolutionize the treatment of psychiatric and neurologic disorders much as the science of microbiology relegated the terror of plagues to history.

Beyond its impact on health and disease, learning the biology of behavior will shake the foundations of our social institutions. Knowing how we learn will change the way we teach. Understanding the roots of criminal behavior will force us to reexamine our penal codes. Finding the biological causes of violence and abuse will tempt us with intrusive methods to reduce their tragic toll. Through medical and surgical means, we will have the imperious ability to exact compliance with behavioral norms. New ways to assess the brain's potential could lead to the rationing of opportunities for education and employment and even change the way that we evaluate and select our leaders. More than ever, the public will need to be well-informed about current science and the choices it presents.

And yet, it is easy to overestimate what is currently known about the brain. When you hear or read reports about specific areas of the brain that "perform" specific functions or "control" certain behaviors, it is important to recognize their hyperbole. They overstate the case. The best we can presently do is to identify *neural correlates,* specific bits of neural activity within the brain that correspond to a particular experience or behavior. Understanding the objective events in the brain that cause you to hear or to see, for example, does not bridge the enormous gap between those neural activities and the grand illusions they produce. Learning the molecular, anatomical, and electrochemical secrets of the brain has not explained the phenomena of subjective experience, but it has put us in a much better position to approach that greater mystery. From our present vantage point, the view of the trail ahead is as exhilarating as the view of the valley from which we have climbed.

Prior to the twentieth century this journey had no reliable

signposts. The brain remained a "black box" permitting only the study of its sensory input and behavioral output. The effects of injury suggested that certain vaguely defined areas of the brain served specific functions, but there were no clues as to how those functions might be carried out. The gelatinous interior of the brain was beyond reckoning.

At the end of the nineteenth century, a new method of staining tissue for the microscope changed the intellectual landscape. Visualizing the brain's stunning internal architecture of branching neurons transformed the conventional view of this seemingly structureless mass. For the first time, the brain was felt to be accessible to study and perhaps even to understanding. At the turn of the century, while L. Frank Baum created apt allegories in his mythical land of Oz, we started down an intriguing road in search of the wizard within us. Like Baum's unforgettable foursome we are traveling down a curious path paved with startling revelations, searching for insights into our nature and for the hidden forces that govern our lives.

We will be joined on this journey by some of the pioneers who first marked this trail. Some are luminaries you have met before, including the Greek anatomist, Galen of Pergamum; the French philosopher and scientist, René Descartes; and America's adopted physicist, Albert Einstein. Others are neuroscientists and Nobel Laureates whom you may be meeting for the first time, such as Stephen Kuffler, John Dowling, Torsten Wiesel, David Hubel, and more. However, we will not follow every step of their mind-bending journey. At the expense of some academic precision we will take a more leisurely trail—complete with steps, handrails, signposts, and occasional benches where we may stop to enjoy the view.

The specific and limited aim of this book is to provide a frame of reference from which to appreciate the exciting advances in neuroscience that appear with increasing frequency on the nightly news. It describes what we know about the brain, how we found out, and what this may mean for the future. It is written for the curious reader whose last scientific reading might have been in a long forgotten classroom and who is now discovering that science is once again a required course in a rapidly changing world. However, I should disclose at the very start, this brief excursion could change the way you think about thinking.

1

Exploring a Recently Discovered Galaxy

Off to See the Wizard

We stand at a turning point of history where we will witness not
only new breakthroughs in weapons of destruction, but a race
for mastery of the sky and the rain, the ocean and the tides,
the far side of space and the inside of men's minds.
—JOHN F. KENNEDY, *accepting the presidential nomination,*
Los Angeles, 1960

I WAS IN MEDICAL SCHOOL in 1960, studying the ingenious
operation and interplay of the organ systems. The nervous
system was a colossal disappointment. Learning the names
of the myriad bumps and fissures of the brain brought me no
closer to understanding its mystery. The only explanation for
what goes on in that magical maze—the organ that governs all
the rest—was that electric impulses travel through it. Neural
signals from one neuron travel across a synapse and stimulate
the receiving branches of the next.

That was about it. And yet, with just a small number of neurons, an ancient sea anemone captured its food and recoiled from its predators. With millions of those communicative cells, a Paleozoic octopus used its eyesight to capture its prey. With billions of neurons, an early human painted murals on the walls of a cave and created lasting images of particular facets of his or her world that held special meaning.

Often a cave painting includes the imprint of the artistic hand that produced it, a signature faithfully replicating every outstretched digit and testifying to the deeply personal origin of that painted metaphor. Those carefully pressed handprints survive as the eloquent expression of a powerful, subjective sense of self, an "I" who looked out from the galaxy of neurons in a skull much like ours and felt the brutal uncertainty as well as the beauty of that ancient world. We do not yet understand how countless, separate nerve cells give rise to that sense of a single and unique being living alone somewhere behind the eyes. Like those early artists, we must still rely on metaphors to describe our personal ecstasy and pain, our individual joy with life and love, our lonely fear of death, and the wrenching, singular despair we suffer from our losses. But we are beginning to understand the intellect behind our high brow. We are learning how the extravagant endowment of neurons behind our bulging, distinctly human forehead enables us to preplan complex movements, to craft tools, to use symbols and language, to enjoy and suffer complex emotions, to create metaphors, and to contemplate the magic that makes us "tick."

From the vast number and complexity of those branching neurons, something enigmatic emerged over the eons, something that seems to have a life of its own. It is capable of introspection and is characterized by consciousness. Like the opening bar of Beethoven's Fifth Symphony, this arresting, forceful emergence appears to stand quite apart from the orchestra where it was given breath; far greater than the sum of its parts and bearing no resemblance to them. Neuroscience is ultimately the study of that powerful presence. With ever more sophisticated tools, we are craning to catch our first glimpse of the mind.

In his recent book, *The Astonishing Hypothesis,* Francis Crick wrote:

> The Astonishing Hypothesis is that "You," your joys and your sorrows, your memories and your ambitions, your sense of personal identity and free will, are in fact no more than the behavior of a vast assembly of nerve cells and their associated molecules. As Lewis Carroll's Alice might have phrased it: You're nothing but a pack of neurons.[1]

But you are not just a collection of nerve cells. In fact, you are not merely a pack of cells of any kind. Universally, in cases where a limb has been deprived of its nervous connections because of injury or disease, patients describe their own arm or leg as an alien object. Although it still contains their flesh and bones replete with all of its blood vessels and nerves, it no longer seems a part of them. The name you give yourself applies directly to the unique pattern of trillions of impulses produced by your one hundred billion neurons. That electrochemical music buzzes from synapse to synapse, from your brain to your toes and back again, reporting momentary alterations in your environment, your body, and the changing relationship between the two.

Your pack of neurons produces a peculiar music that you can hear, feel, smell, taste, and see. The music of the neuron moves you to laughter and tears while it manufactures your memories. Below the level of your conscious awareness, that whispered song also maintains your homeostasis, keeping dozens of mechanical and chemical systems—your heart rate, body temperature, blood pressure, oxygen level, even your mood and disposition—appropriate to your changing environment. The brains of sea slugs, chimpanzees, and human beings each hum with a melody distinguished by its degree of complexity. Each produces a composition dictated by its biology and shaped by evolution. The uniquely human music coursing through your skull can be heard and recorded only with the most delicate of instruments, and these faint signals will lead us on our journey through the brain.

Before embarking on this expedition, it will help to briefly consider where we have been, where we are, and where we are going. Since it is impossible to personally relate to the idea of billions of years, I will ask you to imagine compressing the time line of history so that planet Earth was born one year ago. On this scale, algae began blindly contributing oxygen to the atmosphere nine months ago, oceans spawned jellyfish and sea anemone six months ago, and today—actually, only twelve *minutes* ago—we made our debut on a vibrant, middle-aged planet that is destined to lose its lucky star a little more than a year from now. We have just arrived, and we did so with the greatest number and most complex arrangement of neurons the world has seen.

Just four sensory receptors, each designed to respond to a single flavor—either salty, bitter, sour, or sweet—are able to create a profuse variety of taste sensations by blending their voices and varying the rhythm of their signals. The billions of neurons in your brain constantly vary their tunes and produce a most astonishing repertoire that is heard in every fiber of your being. They create electrical patterns of sufficient complexity to deal adroitly with abstractions; to create contracts, constitutions, symphonies, and shopping malls; and to appreciate the deep, inescapable difference between yesterday and tomorrow.

Because we have so many neurons arranged in such complex networks, signals require a measurable part of a second to travel through them. As a result, we are relatively slow to react when compared with our predecessors. Our movements must appear ponderous to a hummingbird, which, burdened with far fewer neurons, may be able to see the individual beats of its own wings. A fly, with its paucity of neurons, requires practically no time to dodge our clumsy threats. Frogs and birds have a distinct insect-catching advantage over us because of their fewer neurons and much shorter reaction time. However, the time-consuming complexity of the neural connections in our brain, coupled with the incredible dexterity of our hands and voice box, account for our unmatched ingenuity and our unparalleled ability to learn and to teach. With symbols and language, we can transfer new insights from one generation to the next and pool our cumulative knowledge within the cooperative framework of a community.

About ten minutes ago in this one-year history of our planet, we learned to farm and to domesticate animals and just six minutes ago we learned how to write. We have come a long way in twelve minutes but, like hatchling sea turtles racing across the sand toward the relative safety of the surf, we are at a critical point in our infancy. Our survival hinges on our "fitness," an exquisite fit between our biology, our behavior, and the strict demands of an unforgiving yet fragile environment.

In the battle for survival, even with its sluggish habits and poor eyesight, the ancient barnacle is an unqualified champion. Our mobility and our Technicolor view of the world would improve neither its nutrition nor its sustained reproductive success. Different conditions call for different strategies. We, along with birds, have traded away keen smell for sharp vision. We are oblivious to the wealth of information other species can gain from a brief sniff; however, with our noses exposed to molecules swirling far above the ground, such fine olfaction would be more of a distraction than a help. Humans have also traded quickness for cleverness. If our sizes and circumstances were similar, the ungainly frog would fare much better on its lily pad than we would on ours. Due to our peculiar proportions, our erect posture, and the changing nature of our environment, we have evolved with dexterous hands, an agile voice box, billions of neurons in our brain, and, most important of all, a continually growing body of communal knowledge.

These are curious armaments for a vulnerable new species, and we developed them quickly. We had to. Our environment had changed dramatically and abruptly. As the vast forests covering much of Africa swiftly shrank and nearly vanished, most of their quadrapedal, arboreal primates, now suddenly arborless, perished. Some benefited from accidents of mutation, which happened to suit their new circumstances. Seven hours ago on the one-year time line we are using, the first furtive clan of bipedal primates, *Australopithecine anamensis,* began to use their upper limbs primarily for things other than locomotion and support. We learned this by finding Lucy's famous bones in eastern Africa. Only four hours ago, some of Lucy's descendants became skilled tool makers—*Homo habilis*—and two hours later, some of the offspring of *habilis* began to walk with the upright gait and forward-looking posture of *Homo erectus.* Twelve minutes ago, some of the distant descendants of *Homo erectus* began to acquire the familiar, distinctly human countenance of *Homo sapiens*—complete with manual skill, language, and a brain more than twice the size of Lucy's.

In their stable habitat, sharks, jellyfish, and sea anemones have not changed a bit since they first appeared several months ago, yet within only the past few hours, the offspring of *Homo habilis* have acquired brains and bodies far different than their forebears. Of the arboreal primates who were cast out of their shrinking, forested Gardens of Eden, only those able to meet new challenges with brand new behaviors survived to call themselves *Homo sapiens,* the wise ones. If we prove wise enough to survive for another year, when our lucky star runs out of fuel, and migrate like latter-day Noahs from a dying solar system to a new one, history will record that it was during our lifetime, in the last years of the twentieth century of our fledgling calendar, that we took our first steps toward realizing John F. Kennedy's vision of mastering "the far side of space and the inside of men's minds."

FOR MOST OF RECORDED HISTORY, the mind and the far side of space were equally mystical concepts, regarded as the exclusive domains of revered spirits drawn from mythology and theology. In 1748, a French physician, Julien Offroy de La Mettrie, wrote a bold and scholarly treatise proposing that the brain itself, and not an ethereal sprit, was the source of our thoughts.[2] Condemned for blasphemy, he was stripped of his position with the French Guard and was forced to flee to Prussia. Religious dogma held that thought and behavior were supernatural, spiritual phenomena. Although the amorphous brain was believed to passively receive sensations, otherwise, like the spleen and the thymus, the brain appeared to do nothing at all. There was little evidence and even less incentive to connect the lofty mind with the spongy, slimy substance in the skull.

Santiago Ramón y Cajal forever changed the way we view the mind when, about one hundred years ago in Barcelona, he confirmed that the brain contains a huge number of individual nerve cells, a number now estimated to be roughly equal to the number of stars in the Milky Way. Dr. Ramón y Cajal (his family name is usually shortened to Cajal) was enthralled by their microscopic patterns. An accomplished artist as well as a physician, he spent hours copying the shapes of various neurons in exquisite drawings, which are duplicated in today's textbooks. Within their complexity, Cajal found hints of a wonderful order. Similarly shaped neurons are often aligned in neat, parallel rows and each neuron extends branches, numbering from a few to several thousand, toward its neighbors. Refuting the prevalent doctrine that the brain was a continuous, spongy mass, Cajal proposed that each neuron is separate from every other, reaching toward but never actually touching those around it. He postulated that neurons actively communicate with each other, sending messages from the branches of one to the branches of another.[3] No other tissue in the body harbored such an intricate internal organization. Surely this tissue was capable of much more than just the passive reception of sensations.

Fifty years later, anatomists confirmed with the electron microscope that a small gap always separates the branches of one neuron from the next. Physiologists recorded electric impulses passing across this all-important space, and biochemists soon identified the chemicals that selectively transmit electric messages across the synaptic cleft between one neuron and the next.

During the early 1970s, departments of neuroscience began to appear at leading universities around the world. They were as much a product of space age technology as the hand-held calculators and first-generation computers that were beginning to make their appearance on college campuses. Instruments inspired by microengineers at the National Aeronautics and Space Administration (NASA) made it possible for previously unthinkable experiments in neuroanatomy, neuro-physiology, and neurochemistry to be performed quickly and often side by side in the same laboratory. The shoulders and the ideas of scientists from separate disciplines rubbed together as never before and sparked an explosion of research. The sleepy field of neurobiology was transformed, acquiring a new excite-ment, a new prominence, and a new name. Neuroscience was launched.

Clinical neurology benefited almost immediately. Computer scientists and neuroradiologists combined their talent and technology to produce computerized axial tomograms, remark-able X-ray images that showed not only the images of dense bone and cartilage but the three-dimensional, subtle contours of organs as soft as the brain. In 1972, hospitals recognized that this extraordinary benefit was worth its considerable cost and the term CAT scan entered our vocabulary.

Brain surgery could advance only as rapidly as the fanci-ful old drawings and misleading travel brochures collected by prior generations were replaced by accurate road maps. As recently as a few decades ago, the maps of the territory we are now exploring in such detail and the stories told about it were often inaccurate and always unreliable. Lions, tigers, and bears lurked at every bend in the neurosurgical road. Unfor-tunately, even as late as 1969, the true size and the lethal nature of a tumor in the brain of my wife's mother could not be guessed until halfway through a six-hour operation. Times changed quickly. Three years later, computerized axial tomog-raphy would show the exact size, location, and shape of a brain tumor in graphic detail, allowing for early and precise plan-ning of treatment. In 1980, nuclear magnetic resonance, a method used for molecular analysis, was combined with the technique for producing a CAT scan and created a crude image of the brain in about five minutes. By 1986, high-resolution images could be produced in five seconds, and magnetic resonance imaging (MRI) became available for clinical use. The term *nuclear* was dropped from its name because of its negative connotations and because, in fact, the MRI does not use ionizing radiation such as X rays. Its images are formed by energy in the much safer radio frequency range. With negligible risk or discomfort, it is now possible to visualize the living brain as clearly as a laboratory specimen.

Since 1990, two additional imaging techniques have become available that show not only the brain's structure, but its metabolic, biochemical, and functional activity. Positron emission tomography (PET) and functional magnetic resonance imaging (fMRI) allow one not only to visualize a brain tumor prior to surgery, but also to determine whether removing it will interfere with speech, movement, or any other important function. PET scans take from two to four hours to perform and require the injection of a substance that is normally metabolized by brain cells such as glucose, after it has been bound to a briefly radioactive tracer. When the subject performs an assigned task, those areas of the brain that become active are seen in contrasting colors as they metabolize more of the radioactively labeled substance than the surrounding brain tissue. An fMRI scan instead, highlights the increased rate of blood flow that accompanies neural activity in a local area of the brain. This procedure requires no injections or radioactive materials and produces images of extremely high resolution in a few minutes.

To those who first described the squishy, perplexing organ in the skull at the time of Hippocrates in 300 B.C., its most interesting features were its ventricles, the small, fluid-filled spaces at the center of the brain. Five hundred years later, the famous Greek anatomist Galen of Pergamum wrote that it

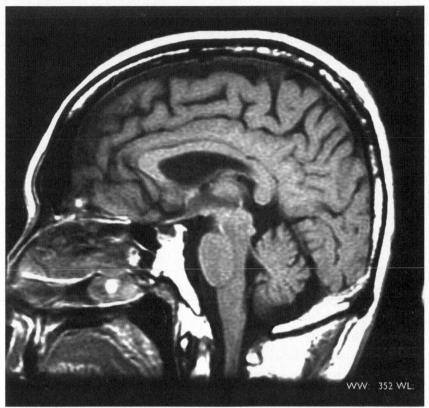

Courtesy of Jerome Barakos, M.D., California Pacific Medical Center, San Francisco

Figure 1.1   Magnetic resonance image of the brain

was in these ventricles that the "animal spirits" reside. With remarkable anatomical detail, he described how vital spirits were inhaled through the lungs and carried through the blood to those hidden chambers in the brain. That concept of inhaled, heavenly spirits animating our earthly bodies remained the core of neuroscience for the next sixteen centuries. Galen's views persisted even after a convincing demonstration in the eighteenth century that electric impulses travel through the nervous system and produce the muscle contractions and the glandular secretions that account for all of our behavior.

You need only draw a deep breath to appreciate the intuitive appeal of Galen's theory. Intuition also led Galen to propose separate sites of action for the rational, vegetative, and animal aspects of our lives. He wrote that rational behavior is mediated through the brain's ventricles, the seat of the rational soul; bodily functions through the liver, the seat of the vegetative soul; and emotional behavior through the heart, the seat of the animal soul. For nearly two thousand years, the amorphous, jellylike tissue of the brain appeared to be nothing more than a natural packing material whose purpose was to cushion the precious contents of the ventricles.

Indeed, like packing paper, the brain seems to have been hurriedly crumpled and stuffed into its tight quarters. If it were possible to spread out only the outer layer of the brain, the cerebral cortex, laying flat its wrinkled folds and fissures, it would cover an area about ten times as large as this page. The wrinkled shape of the cortex appears quite arbitrary except for its clear division into symmetrical right and left halves, each a nearly perfect mirror image of the other. The cerebral cortex, sometimes called the neocortex, has undergone extraordinary and, in evolutionary terms, very recent enlargement. Its crumpled, convoluted appearance is the result of extremely rapid growth, more than doubling in size in the wink of only two million years, within the confines of a rigid, more slowly growing, cranium.

Below the cortex, the human brain bears a striking resemblance to those of much older species. Just as they do in most animals, neurons in the medulla oblongata and pons located at the base of your brain, where it begins to taper into your spinal cord, steadily and reliably regulate your vegetative functions, automatic bodily activity such as your heartbeat and respiration. The brain stem—and not the liver—is the true site of Galen's vegetative soul. Deep within your brain but well above the brain stem, neurons in your pituitary and hypothalamus evolved from cells that enabled your chordate ancestors to sense the chemical perfume of an unseen mate in a distant meadow and to initiate a courtship. Now they sense and regulate the hormones in your blood. They lie deep in the subcortical, central region of the brain, which could be called the seat of your animal soul. This area, truly the heart of your brain, includes several important nuclei that produce and regulate your degree of arousal, the tone and depth of your feelings, and your

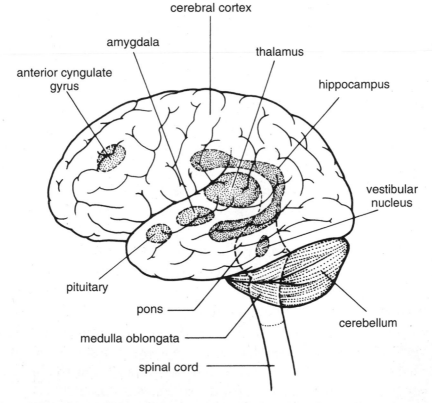

Figure 1.2 Constellations within the brain's galaxy of neurons

19

emotionally directed behavior. The behavior produced in this middle portion of the brain is often labeled instinctual and unthinking because it is less easily modified than the more deliberately planned, finely tuned responses generated in the newly acquired cerebral cortex above it. That massive collection of neurons in the thin outer layer of the brain is the site of Galen's rational soul. It is here in the neocortex that *Homo sapiens* developed the wisdom to modify the instinctual behavior initiated by his inherited, inner brain; to cope with the unfamiliar; to delay gratification when necessary; and to plan, calculate, and survive in an often hostile environment far different from the one for which his body was originally designed.

We will examine this brain specimen only long enough to point out its main features. You will not have to contend with the acrid chemical aroma of the anatomy lab. However, if you are squeamish, you can skip this brief section and meet us later.

In life, the brain is pale pink and amazingly soft. Preserved in formalin, it becomes firm and loses its color. The *cerebral cortex,* the thin, vulnerable, convoluted, outer layer of the brain, turns gray as do several areas in its interior, its *nuclei* and *ganglia.* The *gray matter,* packed with billions of neurons and their network of short branches, has the mushy consistency of cooked oatmeal. The rest of the brain, the *white matter,* is a collection of long, insulated *axons,* outgoing branches of neurons that connect various parts of the brain to each other, to the spinal cord, and to the rest of the body. The white matter owes its color to myelin, a glistening, lipid, insulating material wrapped around those long axons. Myelin also gives the white matter its more substantial consistency, which varies from that of firm Jell-O in some areas to the considerable stiffness of modeling clay in others. Looking at the brain provides no clues as to what it does or how it does it.

The brain's functioning—and yours—depends on preserving delicate lines of communication. Even the slightest deformation of the fragile gray matter destroys the critical connections of its billions of neurons, interrupting the transmission of its signals and disturbing the harmony of its faint, electrochemical music. Loss of myelin in the white matter, as occurs in the disease of multiple sclerosis, hampers the transmission of signals down the brain's longer axons.

As is the case in most organizations, the majority of the brain's personnel are support staff. Each neuron is surrounded by ten to fifty *glial cells,* which make up the bulk of the brain. Lacking the exciting executive functions of the neuron, they take a backseat in terms of interesting research. Glial cells serve the neuron in several ways. They provide structural support, insulate longer neural branches with myelin to speed electric signals down their axons, maintain nutrition, aid in waste removal, and even lay down the markers that lead the branches of a developing neuron to its proper destination. A study of Albert Einstein's brain showed that he may have had an overabundance of glial cells, and the significance of this finding awaits a full explanation. Glial cells have recently been discovered to exchange electric signals with neurons, and it would not be surprising to find that they have important, still unsuspected functions.[4]

The brain's most guarded secret is how the signals of the neuron are transformed into the epiphenomena of our subjective experience, how electric impulses become the familiar stuff of life. Glial cells are certainly ideally situated to appreciate the neuron's electrical performance. Although there is as yet no solid evidence to support this speculative notion, it is tempting to wonder if the glial cell is where this mysterious translation of the neurons' electric signals into recognizable

21

mental phenomena occurs, and whether this translation occurred more easily for Albert Einstein because he had more glial cells than most of us.

The brain's secrets and its vulnerable, precious collection of cells is encased in a rigid skull lined by shock-absorbing membranes and cushioned by a clear fluid, the cerebrospinal fluid. This liquid fills the ventricles, percolates through the outer membranes that surround the brain, and a tiny trickle seeps into the brain tissue to bathe the neurons and glial cells. Cerebrospinal fluid (CSF) is filtered out of the blood much like the fluid that bathes cells elsewhere in your body, but it passes through a filter so selective that it is called the *blood-brain barrier*. Only small molecules, such as those of oxygen and glucose, pass easily from the blood into the CSF. Larger molecules are kept out of the brain unless they are shaped specifically to pass through this formidable blockade. The molecules of only a relatively few drugs are able to pass through the blood-brain barrier to influence the function of the brain.

In spite of all we have learned since the second century, Galen's legacy is still embedded in our vocabulary. Depending on the degree to which it is rational or emotional, we describe our behavior as coming either from the head or from the heart. A forced, polite smile is easy to distinguish from one that comes "from the heart," and it is difficult to fake the latter. A courteous smile, produced on demand, begins in the newly evolved prefrontal cortex and involves only the voluntary contraction of the muscle in your cheek. The unmistakable warmth of a genuine smile, one triggered by true emotion, appears when the muscles around your eyes add their revealing contribution. This splendid co-contraction occurs as an involuntary response to neurons in the anterior cyngulate gyrus in the "older," limbic portion of your brain, neurons that respond only to prescribed sets of stimuli.[5] Their neural activity can be initiated voluntarily only with great difficulty and considerable acting talent.

It is as though three brains inhabit your skull. In order of evolutionary age, and going from the base of the brain to the top, the first consists of the vegetative, nonthinking brain stem with its autonomic nervous system. This part of the brain maintains your vital signs—the pulse, temperature, and blood pressure that are among the first entries made in your hospital chart, right after the name of your insurance carrier. Above this basal portion of your brain is the larger, animal brain, which orchestrates your emotive, instinctual behavior. In the head versus heart dilemmas you are forever debating, this is the voice of your heart. The genuine smile originates here. So does the mania and the depression of bipolar disease; the uncontrollable, ritualized behavior and fixed ideas of obsessive compulsive disorder; and the desperate, suicidal impulses of major depression. Crowning this hotbed of emotion, this generator of intense feelings, is the cognitive cortex—the wrinkled, recently evolved rational brain that decides when it may truly be appropriate to feel depressed or manic, to perform a ritual, or to stay rigidly focused on a single idea. Your cerebral cortex lets you know when a smile would be in your immediate best interest.

⚙ ⚙

THE SOURCE OF ANY SMILE, genuine or not, remained a complete mystery until quite recently and it is worth taking a moment to review how we came to guess the brain's central, creative role in producing your behavior. In the year 1504, Gregor Reisch published an encyclopedia, *The Margarita Philosophica,*

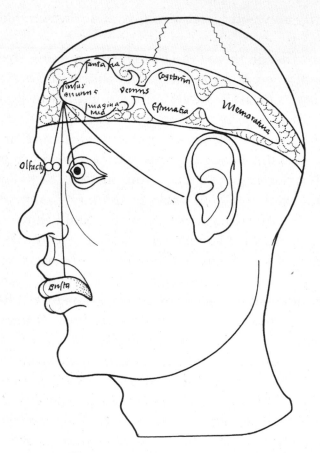

Figure 1.3 The brain in 1504

which is still prized for its elaborate woodcut prints. One of the illustrations in Reisch's book beautifully depicts the state of neuroscience at the height of the Renaissance. The printing press, a novelty only fifty years earlier, was creaking into general use, spreading stories of the New World to Europeans who were just beginning to enjoy tobacco, and firing their imaginations with the powerful idea that one could circumnavigate the planet. Leonardo da Vinci and Michelangelo had broken the strong taboos surrounding the study of human anatomy. Western art and science were once again exploring nature with rational principles abandoned for more than a thousand years.[6]

In the sixteenth century as in the second, the mind was envisioned as a supernatural spirit swimming in a special fluid, separate from the body and immune to the laws of the natural world. Based on resurrected ancient Greek writings, Reisch portrayed mental functions as taking place not in the brain's tissue, but within three distorted renditions of the brain's ventricles. The largest cavity in the center of Reisch's cutaway view of the head is described as the seat of *thought and judgment,* the rear cavity is labeled as the seat of *memory,* and the cavity near the front of the brain, drawn with lines connecting it with the eyes, nose, mouth, and ears, is labeled *common sensory.* It is especially interesting that Reisch also described the *common sensory* cavity as the seat of *fantasy and imagination.* Although his anatomy proved wrong, his intuitive notion—that internal imagery arises in the same location where sensory perception occurs—was correct. It was confirmed by positron emission tomography almost five hundred years later. The areas of the brain that become active on a PET scan when you experience a sensation light up again when you later close your eyes and imagine that experience.

Fifty years after Reisch's encyclopedia was printed, René Descartes published a comprehensive description of the human body that became the authoritative owner's manual for the next three centuries. Descartes combined his mastery of the mechanical principles governing water-driven clockworks and other hydraulic devices, which were the high-tech marvels of his day, with elaborate anatomical drawings based on the writings of Galen. From the 1550s to the 1850s, those detailed drawings gave credence to Descartes's theory that fluid alternately fills and empties antagonistic pairs of muscles to produce the body's movements with their reciprocal, leverlike action. His, too, was a dualistic construction, separating mind from body, but he no longer evoked the brain's ventricles as the reservoirs of the soul. Descartes proposed that the engine animating this hydraulic machine is a supernatural spirit exerting its influence through the pineal gland at the anatomical center of the brain.

The concept that the mind and body are separate was strongly sanctioned by religious leaders and went largely unquestioned until 1748, when the French physician Julien Offroy de La Mettrie wrote his scandalous and ill-fated treatise, *L'Homme machine,* challenging Galen, Descartes, and the Church. He dared, at the cost of his career, to seriously propose that the source of our thoughts was the brain alone.

In an experiment repeated in countless biology classes, Luigi Galvani demonstrated in 1791 that a frog muscle contracts when stimulated by electricity. That twitch of an amphibian leg was the first evidence of the true nature of our animal spirits. Gradually and grudgingly, scientists began to concede that, while the heart pumps blood and the kidneys make urine, the brain produces electric impulses. Yet even when the electrical nature of nerve impulses was confirmed by Emil du Bois-Reymond in 1843, very few were willing to give up the ghost of Galen and believe that electrical activity in the brain was responsible for "higher" mental function.

Like the exiled Dr. La Mettrie, the German anatomist Franz Gall again challenged the dualistic concept of mind and body in Austria in 1802—perhaps more colorfully, but with no more success. Gall collected the skulls of criminals and the busts of famous men and correlated the bumps in those skulls with the mental faculties that were prominent in the lives of their owners. From this data, he drew a detailed map identifying the particular areas of the cerebral cortex, which he proposed were responsible for each of twenty-seven distinct

26

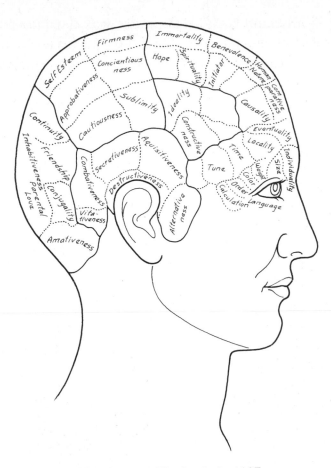

Figure 1.4 The brain in 1807

mental functions. His theory, too, was completely abhorrent to the Church and found no support in the scientific community. Gall was expelled from Austria in 1807 and from the prestigious French Academy of Science in 1808.

Gall's blasphemous proposal gave birth to the popular folly of phrenology, interpreting a personality from bumps on the head. Phrenology would persist as a favorite parlor game well into the next century. In an age of chaperones, when physical contact of any kind between the sexes was considered risqué, phrenology provided a rare opportunity for proper ladies and gentlemen to caress the contours of each other's cranium, comparing it with a copy of Gall's chart and pretending to look for clues to behavior and temperament. Phrenology was used both for fun and profit. Itinerant phrenologists could be found at most carnivals, department store openings, or anywhere a crowd had gathered or where someone would pay to create one. With elaborate charts and great enthusiasm, they would espouse the wonders of this new "science" and charge a modest fee to "read" your skull. As phrenology began to compete with fortune-telling, its popularity reflected a growing but naive fascination with the brain.

Then, quite suddenly in the mid 1800s, two patients, one on either side of the Atlantic Ocean, forced a more serious look at the correlation between behavior and specific regions of the brain. Careful clinical observation began to replace intuition as the preferred guide into that unknown territory. The first of these cases was the now-famous, nearly fatal accident of Phineas Gage, the foreman of a railroad construction crew working near Cavendish, Vermont, in 1848.

While tamping down the blasting powder for a dynamite charge, Gage unwittingly provided a compelling argument for the brain's role in shaping behavior. A spark prematurely ignited his powder and blasted an inch-thick metal tamping rod through his left cheek and out through the top of his head. Amazingly, although he lost an eye, within two months Gage could walk, talk, and function normally. His behavior, however, was no longer that of the affable, reliable Phineas Gage who had earned the respect of his friends, family, and co-workers. He was now a foulmouthed, irresponsible, ill-mannered, habitual liar. His physician, Dr. John Harlow, was so impressed by this personality change that his clinical records contain this radical conclusion: "The damage to the frontal lobe of the brain has destroyed the equilibrium between his intellectual faculties and animal propensities."

Whether Gage's brain injury had actually altered his "faculties and propensities" was debated for over a century. When Phineas Gage died during an epileptic seizure thirteen years later, Dr. Harlow persuaded his family to donate his skull to medical research and it was preserved in the Warren Medical Museum at Harvard University. One hundred and thirty-three years later, armed with computerized models and modern imaging techniques, Hanna and Antonio Damasio, neuroscientists at the University of Iowa, settled the question. They pinpointed the site of the damage to Gage's brain and determined that the tamping rod had destroyed the ventromedial region in the underbelly of the left frontal lobe. Damage to this general area has been documented to cause exactly the same personality changes described in Dr. Harlow's records of the unfortunate Phineas Gage.

The case of Phineas Gage raised enough questions and controversy that, by 1861, the medical community was ready to seriously consider another case where brain damage was claimed to be the cause of a behavioral change. Dr. Paul Broca provided convincing evidence that the brain was indeed the source of higher functions with his report of a patient in Paris who, as a result of a stroke, developed "motor aphasia," the inability to speak. Although the man knew what he wanted to say and was even able to write the words, the sounds that he uttered were unintelligible even to himself. Upon the patient's death, Dr. Broca performed an autopsy that revealed a lesion in the middle part of the frontal lobe on the left side of the brain, an area known today as Broca's motor area for speech. In a statement designed to directly challenge established scientific and religious dogma, he is said to have proclaimed that "we speak with the left hemisphere." The next few years were to prove him right.

During the carnage of the Prusso-Danish and American civil wars in the 1860s, brain lesions were sadly becoming prolific instructors of neurology. In all cases in which Broca's area was damaged, motor aphasia was the result. It also became obvious that injury to one side of the brain causes paralysis on the opposite side of the body. The jurisdiction of the brain is divided between its two halves and it is crossed. The eyes respect this division and go one better. The nerve fibers from each retina, the light-capturing layer at the back of the eye, split on their way through the brain. The fibers from the half of the retina closest to your nose cross to the opposite side. Each half of the brain, therefore, connects with only one half of *each* eye. If you draw a vertical line down the middle of your field of view, everything to the right of that line is seen only by the left side of your brain. If your left occipital lobe (see Fig. 1.6) is damaged, the right half of your visual world disappears.

In 1875, a young German neurologist, Carl Wernicke, discovered a new dimension in the unfolding complexity of the brain. He was the first to propose that a complex behavior might be the result of a *neural circuit,* a specific path that signals follow through the brain. He described a lesion in the left temporal lobe that produced sensory aphasia, the inability to understand spoken words or to organize them coherently. Wernicke suggested, correctly, that neural signals are transmitted from the ears to this area, now called Wernicke's area, in the left temporal lobe where they are organized into language, and travel from there to Broca's area in the left frontal lobe where they activate the motor control of speech. Wernicke's concept of distinctive patterns of signal transmission through the brain provided the first rational approach to understanding how the brain works.

The stunning notion of such an elegant interplay of specific

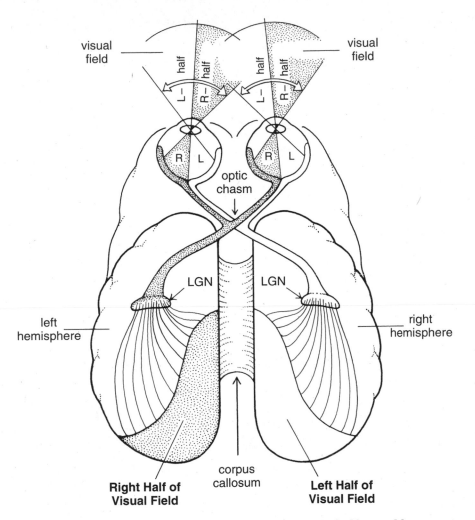

Figure 1.5 Each half of the brain sees only half a world

functional "centers" rekindled the effort to complete a meaningful map of the human brain. A search was begun for the brain's
blueprint, for more evidence of a hidden order in the unusual
anatomy of the brain. By 1909, Korbinian Brodmann, using both
monkeys and humans, had identified fifty-two areas of the brain
that showed a correlation with a particular function.

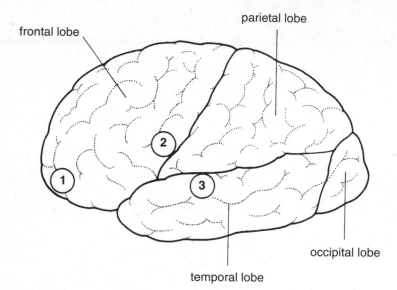

1. Ventromedial area for Phineas Gage's "propensities"
2. Broca's motor area for motor control of speech
3. Wernicke's area for interpretation of speech

Figure 1.6   The brain in 1875

Brain mapping became the primary focus of neurology, and it took a huge leap forward during the 1940s, when Dr. Wilder Penfield and his colleagues in Montreal stimulated the brains of awake patients undergoing neurosurgery. Because the brain is devoid of pain-sensitive receptors, Dr. Penfield and his associates were able to stimulate accessible areas of the brain with a tiny electric current and record their patients' reactions during surgery. As each area was stimulated, they noted whether the patient heard a sound, felt a touch on the left foot, moved the right thumb, etc. Their findings solidified the concept of localized, sensory and motor areas and produced much more reliable maps of the human brain showing the location of numerous functional centers.[7]

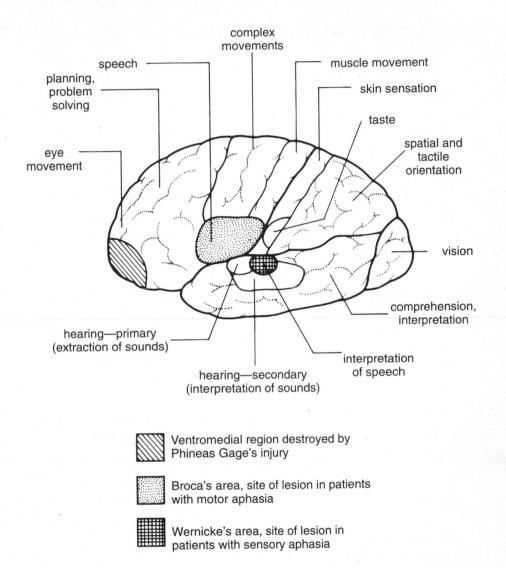

Figure 1.7   The brain in 1945

By 1950, it became clear that things were not so simple. Clinical cases began to suggest that the centers for brain function are far from autonomous. For example, lesions quite remote from the centers for language or vision severely interfered with these functions. Some physicians and biologists began to suspect that there might be very little intrinsic organization to the brain at all, that all of its parts might be equipotential and interchangeable. It took some interesting detective work to learn that the brain is neither a collection of autonomous centers nor is it a single, uniform, multifunctional system. It is a most curious blend of the two. The first clues came from the operating room.

In a bold attempt to prevent the spread of epileptic seizures from one half of the cortex to the other, surgeons severed the narrow bridge of fibers that connects them, the corpus callosum. Happily, aside from alleviating their seizures, "splitting the brains" of these patients seemed at first not to affect them in the least. The millions of fibers connecting the two halves of the cerebral cortex seemed to be completely expendable.

This procedure was abandoned when, over the next decades, a series of experiments with these patients showed that these "expendable" connections between the two halves of the cortex in fact have a most surprising purpose. Normally, your two hemispheres are in constant, silent communication with each other through the corpus callosum, and the richness of your life depends on the continuous conversation between them. Each half of your brain perceives and relates to the world independently—and each in its own, distinct way. Severing the corpus callosum prevents them from sharing their separate views.[8]

As you read the following experiment, remember that each half of your brain has jurisdiction over only one-half of each eye. When you stare at the center of a screen, an image flashed on its left half will be seen only by the right half of your brain. In a now famous experiment, the picture of a spoon was flashed on the left half of a screen in front of a "split-brain" patient, a patient who had undergone surgical splitting of the corpus callosum. When asked what he saw, the patient curiously reported seeing nothing. Although the right hemisphere had seen the spoon, as Broca pointed out, "we speak with the left hemisphere." The patient's left brain had, in fact, not seen the image on the screen, and it said so.

The patient was then asked to reach under a cloth with his left hand and choose out of several objects the one whose image had been flashed on the screen. The right half of the patient's brain, which had seen the spoon, recognized its shape in his left hand. The patient held up the spoon even though he had just reported seeing nothing on the screen. When asked why he had selected this object, the patient (or rather the patient's left hemisphere, which speaks) confabulated that it was a mere guess and let the matter drop. The patient did not seem in the least perplexed or puzzled by his deliberate selection of the spoon. His left brain could not explain it. His right brain was content with having seen and then having selected the spoon from under the cloth and was not aware that the left brain had reported not seeing it. No part of his brain was aware of the contradiction. With the fibers of the corpus callosum severed and the two halves of the brain unable to share their information, two conflicting sets of knowledge existed side by side and the patient had no recognition of the disparity. The term *split-brain patient* was much more apt than was at first appreciated. Further experiments with these patients, who by now had achieved semicelebrity status, showed that the left hemisphere processes information more quickly than the right. The faster-acting left brain controls complex voluntary movement and calculations, while more artistic and intuitive functions are performed better by the right half of the brain.

Like those enthralled with phrenology a century ago, we are still intrigued by the prospect of identifying the anatomical source of each temperament and behavior. The difference is that now we have some reliable insights. Severing the corpus callosum disclosed that the two halves of your brain behave differently. As you write a letter the old fashioned way, with pen and paper, you will notice that while your writing hand performs its series of complex movements, your other hand is not idle. Your left hand (if you are right-handed), guided by your right brain, stabilizes the paper and makes the continuous adjustments necessary to keep it positioned properly to accept the next word at the proper angle and location.

Whether you are throwing a spear or a spiral pass, chipping a rock or using a fountain pen, one hand is typically used to make adjustments for balance, efficiency, and symmetry while the other makes rapid, deft movements calculated to be both forceful and precise.

The left hemisphere in almost everyone, even in most left-handed persons, is the *dominant hemisphere.* It excels in performing rapid and precise computations and in directing fine, repetitive movements. These skillful movements are internally driven, they are rehearsed, memorized and require very little sensory monitoring once they begin. The *nondominant hemisphere* deals with gestalt. The right hemisphere directs stabilizing, orienting, and corrective movements that are spontaneous and externally driven. They are based on perceptions of patterns, spatial configuration, and on a sense of the whole seen separately from its parts. Because they are unplanned and unfold as they are improvised, they can be modified in mid-course.

One interesting and plausible explanation for this lateralization of the brain is based on the observation that it probably occurred during the few hours (beginning two million years ago in real time) while Lucy's offspring *Homo habilis* developed the talent for the skillful use of tools.[9] The left brains of *Homo habilis* acquired the additional neural circuitry required for those deft and purposeful movements, causing a slight asymmetry of their skulls. Skills such as accurate spear throwing, wood carving, and stone chipping require a period of practice and repetition before the muscles and the neurons that perform such feats achieve a reproducible level of success. It would be logical for novices to use the same hand each time they practice and to imitate the hand choice of their teachers. It is not known whether the lateralization of the brain preceded or followed *Homo habilis*'s early use of tools; however, once the left hemisphere developed the ability to direct quick, repetitive, practiced movements, the stage was set for this talent to also express itself in the fine motor control of the lips, tongue, and larynx and hasten the development of speech and language.

Specialized neural connections in the dominant half of the brain may have been the product—or cause—of our ancestors' emerging dexterity. In either case, the left hemisphere developed an enlarged area at its front end with neural circuitry specially suited for throwing, pounding, and carving, for calculating trajectories, speed, distance, force and, later, for symbol recognition and language. It may have done so at the expense of other networks designed for spatial orientation and that lend themselves to complex pattern recognition, music, art, and intuition—networks that remain better preserved in the right hemisphere.

The rich variety of human behavior relies heavily on the subtle difference between the two sides of the brain. The virtuosity of a concert pianist requires more than the practiced precision of the left hemisphere to execute the notes. True artistry lies in the special ability of the right hemisphere to recognize gestalt, to view the whole composition separately from its parts and to create a rendition that bears the personal stamp of the artist. The right hemisphere makes spontaneous adjustments to shape the speed and force of the fingers and fit their actions to a unique interpretation of the total piece of music, rich with emotive subtlety.

Today, the high hopes raised by increasingly precise maps of the brain have been dashed by the realization that the brain has less regard for its own anatomical regions than we do. We can now trace the paths of neural circuits quite precisely, and they often disregard the compartments that we have drawn. Shaping spear tips, solving quadratic equations, or playing a Chopin sonata each require the coordinated activity of neurons in nearly every part of your brain.

Every age has used contemporary analogies to imagine how the brain "works." Our grandparents pictured signals traveling along nerves and through the brain like Morse code clicking along telegraph wires, or messages in metal cylinders hissing through pneumatic tubes between a department store's central office and distant clerks at their registers. Now we have computers on our minds and tend to think of the brain as though it processes information, records perceptions, and plays back memories as if they were digital bits on a hard drive or a compact disc. However, this completely ignores the enigmatic ways that the brain interweaves input and output. As you will see in Chapter 2, perceptions are as much a product of the brain as of the environment. Neuroscience is forcing us to rethink the relationship of physical and perceptual reality in ways that may surprise you.

It is true that some rudimentary aspects of the brain's magic can be reproduced by machines and, in Chapter 10, we will explore how "neural network" computers modeled on the brain's unique parallel circuitry can even beat chess champions at their own game. It is tempting to speculate that reproducing the complexity of the brain's circuitry on a silicon chip could create an R2D2 or a 3CPO with all of the intelligence, feelings, and foibles of Luke Skywalker or Princess Leia. However, these *Star Wars* creations do not account for the living, breathing biology and molecular chemistry of the neuron. The brain is not your typical electric circuit. It is not even a complex, computerlike series of microcircuits. It is not that simple.

Electric signals traverse your brain through neural circuits that are unlike any electrical circuits that may come immediately to your mind. Currents of neural signals flow throughout the brain in ever-changing patterns and the routes they take—their neural circuits—vary from moment to moment. Signals diverge from one location to arrive at many others. They converge from many areas toward one. They travel in loops to change the output from their source. They take parallel paths, each of which can also converge and diverge. And along each path, a distinctive melody is produced by multitudes of molecules, by single neurons, and by vast neural ensembles. Perhaps it is not unreasonable to suggest that this pattern of signals coursing from neuron to neuron is the melody of life. Neural signals are not confined to your head, but travel through your nerves to every part of your body. In a very real sense, your mind extends to your fingertips. The sensory signals converging toward the brain are as important in determining your behavior as the action-producing signals going the other way.

Serious efforts to localize schizophrenia, attention deficit disorder, musical ability, or even Phineas Gage's personality change to one specific area of the cortex, in more than just a general way, are almost always foiled by the rich and surprisingly extensive communication of neurons. It is more accurate and useful to appreciate that some areas simply contribute more significantly to a particular task than others. For example, even though almost every part of the brain and spinal cord is involved in some way with regulating your gait, the tremors and the rigid, shuffling gait of patients with Parkinson's disease are, in fact, caused by the malfunctioning of a tiny group of cells named for their dark color, the substantia nigra. These cells are nestled within a pair of subcortical islands of gray matter, the basal ganglia, in the older, deeper region of the brain. Not far from the basal ganglia are three other small areas of special interest: a group of cells in the *amygdala* contributes reflexively to your emotions; a second group in the *hippocampus* stores memories; and a third, the *thalamus,* is the gateway for virtually all of your sensations and directs impulses generated by each of your sensory neurons to its appropriate area in the cortex.

Before turning to the contributions of individual areas of the brain, it is important to emphasize the point that no area, and no neuron, works alone—and none is indispensable. Moment by moment, in healthy communication with every other, each neuron produces signals that strive to create an appropriate response to every change in your environment, to match your current situation with behavior that will maximize your chances for survival. Even the exact location of a neuron seems not to matter very much. So long as its branches can reach appropriate neighbors and it is able to send and receive signals, it contributes to a delicately embroidered pattern of impulses that is distinctly recognizable as you.

While the shape of your bones, muscles, heart, and stomach are dictated by their function, molded by the physical forces they encounter, the brain would probably work just as well if it had evolved into the shape of a Tootsie Roll or a Rubik's Cube. The shape of the brain is a clue to its evolutionary history, but says nothing of its function. It appears to be completely arbitrary that you speak with the posterior-inferior portion of the third convolution of the left frontal lobe, that you react to danger with your almond-shaped amygdala, and catalogue memories with your sea-horse–shaped hippocampus—areas that we will visit later. Each section of the brain's orchestra was shoved into its present location for reasons having nothing to do with function and everything to do with such mundane considerations as the constraints of available space and which neurons got there first. Neurons in all of the brain's lumps and bumps contribute to a single, complex musical composition. Learning their locations tells us where to best hear the woodwinds, the brass, or the strings, and it allows the clinician to correlate symptoms with the most likely location of a disease or injury. However, the real secrets of brain function are to be found not in its rather arbitrary anatomy, but in the critical shapes of its molecules, in the patterns of its branching neurons, in the routes of its transmitted signals, and in its combined electrochemical musical score.

The work of your brain takes place on the imperceptible scale of *nanometers* (billionths of a meter) and *milliseconds* (thousandths of a second). We are discovering its secrets because we are developing the ability to fathom those dimensions. We are finally able to describe the details of its electrical activity, its molecular machinery, the inherited set of instructions coded in its genetic material, and the surprising effects that your personal encounters with your environment have on that inherited blueprint. To continue this incredible voyage requires that you shrink to an invisible size.

2

Stardust and the
Music of the Neuron

Impulses and How They Move You

REAL PROGRESS IN UNDERSTANDING the brain began very quietly. Not many had heard of the two recipients of the Nobel Prize in 1952, Andrew Huxley and Alan Hodgkin, and even fewer appreciated the significance of their discoveries. Even those who knew about their years spent studying the neuron of a giant squid believed it to be an obscure, purely academic exercise. The practical importance of the Huxley-Hodgkin equations derived from those experiments is only now beginning to be fully realized. These two scientists asked not where the work of the brain takes place, but how.

Answering this question required maps drawn on a much smaller scale than those traced by Wilder Penfield on the surface of the brain. Huxley and Hodgkin inspired a small band of neurophysiologists and cellular biologists to begin charting a course into the microcosm of the neuron. Armed with new techniques for analyzing a single living cell, they set out on an audacious search for nothing less than the spark of life, the source of the "animal spirit" that Galen had described nearly two thousand years before. Galen probably would have dismissed their remarkable findings as far too fanciful to command serious consideration.

Our nervous systems run on battery power, and fortunately, our batteries are included. They were passed down to us by our earliest, single-celled ancestors. Dissolved in our bodies as in theirs are the electrically charged ions of the salts found in the oceans where life began, ions of sodium (Na^+), potassium (K^+), calcium (Ca^{++}), chloride (Cl^-), magnesium (Mg^{++}), and others— particles that were forged in the explosions of ancient stars. Every living cell, by pumping certain of these ions through its outer membrane, acquires a negative electrical charge on the inside of its membrane, a *resting membrane potential*. Energy borrowed from the stars distinguishes a living cell from a dead one.

During the 1950s, as jet planes and television began shrinking our world, the electron microscope dramatically expanded it. This rather complicated camera uses electrons rather than light to photograph its tiny subjects, and it soon became as much a trademark of the serious laboratory as the magnifying glass had been for Sherlock Holmes. Viewing a miniature Earth through an ordinary microscope, New York City would appear as only a vague smudge. The additional magnification of the electron microscope would bring into focus its buildings and even the rough outlines of its bustling inhabitants. The electron microscope revealed the details of a strange, new landscape and showed us that, although the cell wall is not a simple membrane, it holds a simple secret.

Surrounding each of your cells is a double membrane perforated by oddly shaped tubes or channels, each of which is a tubular molecule of protein through which ions continuously enter and leave the cell. Some of these ion channels behave like

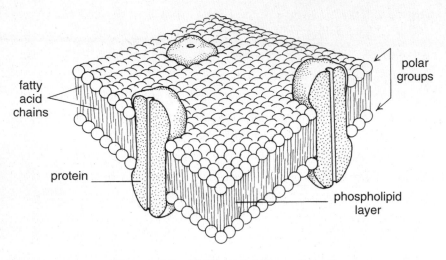

Figure 2.1 (Schematic) The cell wall

bouncers at the door of a saloon, expelling unwanted sodium ions (Na^+) and admitting favored potassium ions (K^+). As if motor driven, they operate around the clock, checking the ID of every ion passing through and controlling the nature and number of admissions. Positively charged ions always escort negative ions through these passages, but Huxley and Hodgkin proved that fewer negative ions leave with sodium (Na^+) than accompany potassium (K^+) into the cell. The resulting surplus of negative ions inside the cell creates the resting membrane potential. Every point along the cell wall becomes a storage battery with its negative pole on the inside and its positive pole on the outside of that vital membrane.[1] A cell's life, and yours, depends on the continuous operation of *sodium-potassium pumps* in the walls of your cells. These miniature gatekeepers are kept running by a complex set of chemical reactions which, for their ultimate source of energy, burn sugar (combining it with oxygen) to produce carbon dioxide and water.

The size of the resting membrane potential varies from cell

Outside of Cell:
High concentration of sodium (NA+)

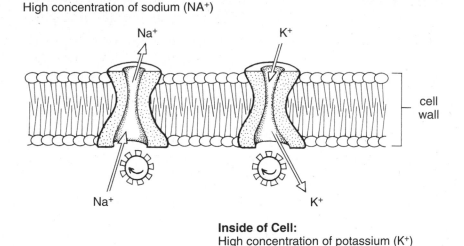

Figure 2.2 (Schematic) Sodium-potassium pumps

to cell, but in a neuron it is about twice as large as in most others, equal to about one-twentieth the charge of a typical penlight battery. The invention of the electron microscope allowed us to see how the neuron activates its resting membrane potential in order to animate us. The neuron is an *excitable cell*. It has the unique ability to cause momentary changes in its resting membrane potential and to produce electric impulses. You tick because it ticks. Its impulses produce your impulses. Imagine trying to convince Galen that your spark of life is borrowed from bits of stardust, flung eons ago from dying suns exploding far beyond our own, and now dissolved in the substance of your body. This seems no less whimsical than his intuitive notion of inhaled, heavenly spirits.

In 1935, the strange electrical behavior of the neuron diverted the attention and the professional life of Andrew Huxley, whose already famous half-brother Aldous Huxley had published the novel *Brave New World* three years earlier. Andrew had just entered Cambridge University on a scholarship and was planning a career in physics, when he became intrigued by the work of an older student. Alan Hodgkin had begun experimenting with the neuron of a giant squid, a neuron so enormous that it was possible to insert a glass pipette into its axon and carefully study its chemical and electric responses to neural stimulation.

Hodgkin and Huxley proved what a pivotal role two particular bits of stardust, sodium, and potassium play in our lives. At precisely timed intervals during the course of the neuron's excitation, they carefully measured the concentrations of those ions on each side of its cell wall and then tediously solved by hand, the thousands of equations necessary to correlate those measurements with the electrical activity of the neuron. That work put the science into neuroscience; it quantified the electrochemical basis of our behavior and it is the platform upon which current brain research stands.

The huge axons of a giant squid led us to recognize the genius of the neuron, its ability to create small shifts in the flow of ions across its membrane. This electric restlessness has altered the course of natural history. The evolution of the neuron was nothing less than the arrival of a new agent for change in the universe. The neuron's excitability caused mobile, sensate creatures to burrow and nest, to alter the earth's topography, to design and use machines, to duplicate the thermonuclear fury of the stars and even to navigate among them. Hodgkin and Huxley set us on a solid path to learn how this cell's simple ability to direct the flow of ions could make possible all of the events that make life interesting and unpredictable. They showed electron microscopists and cellular biologists where to focus their attention and they taught us "where the action is" in the seemingly sedentary brain.

The neuron owes its remarkable talent to specialized openings in its membrane, *gated ion channels* that are unique to the neuron. Just as the tones of a wind instrument are formed by the flow of air through its key stops and valves, the electric signals of the neuron are produced by controlling the flow of ions through these gated openings in its cell wall. Opening and closing the gates in these extraordinary channels produces localized changes in its resting membrane potential. As brief and as faint as these voltage changes may be, they account for your precious awareness of the world, your ability to respond to it—and to change it.

The irregular, tubular molecules of protein that form the gated channels in the wall of the neuron are small, about a billionth of a meter across. For them, the half-inch distance across your fingertip is, on a relative scale, equivalent to your distance from the moon. It is on this tiny scale that these potentially earthshaking impulses are produced. The names and diagrams of these ion channels and the equations that describe their actions quickly fill blackboards and journals, but what they do is surprisingly simple. They open and they close.

The complex functions of the brain begin with only two kinds of gated channels on the surface of a neuron, distinguished by the switch that opens them. *Voltage-gated* channels swing open when they sense a local change in the membrane potential in their immediate area. *Chemically gated* channels open only in response to a particular molecule, either a *transmitter* molecule acting from outside the cell, or a *chemical messenger* molecule acting from within the cell. However, there are dozens of chemicals that can act as transmitters and chemical messengers and there are receptors sensitive to each of them. Therein lies the incredible sophistication of the neuron.

The intelligence of the neuron lies in your DNA, the inherited instruction manual in the nucleus of each cell. About one-third of your genes carry specific directions only for the neuron, dictating what kind of channels it will make, where it will put them, and what kind of receptors each will have. That, in turn, dictates which stimuli the neuron will ignore and to which it will respond. However, many of those instructions include the word "if." Many of those genes simply sit and wait to see *if* a particular set of circumstances comes to pass. They do nothing generation after generation until a situation arises that they recognize as their cue to turn on. Only then, in response to a pre-arranged signal, do they sculpt the particular protein that they were designed to assemble out of the chemicals floating in the surrounding cellular soup. For example, *if* a neuron is overstimulated by cocaine, it will take protective action. Within minutes of exposure to cocaine, a gene (named c-fos) recognizes its cue, turns on, and stops the production of those particular receptors that are sensitive to that drug.[2] The addict, unaware of that intelligent cellular strategy, notices only that he needs more of the drug to achieve its exhilarating effect, and ignores this increasing tolerance at his peril.

Remarkably, each ion channel in the wall of the neuron, whether voltage gated or chemically gated, will admit only a particular ion because of the size and shape of its opening and the peculiar affinities of its molecule. Those that admit sodium (Na^+) have an immediate effect. As soon as sodium channels are opened, additional sodium ions flow into the cell decreasing the resting potential in the immediate area, *depolarizing* it and exciting nearby voltage-gated channels. These local voltage changes spread down a neuron's axon the way that football fans send a "wave" along a stadium's benches, each voltage-gated ion channel getting its cue from the one next to it. As each one

Outside of Cell

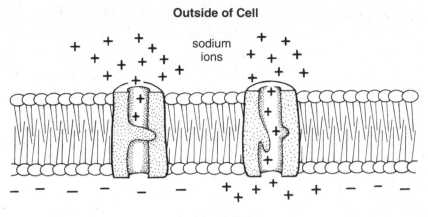

Inside of Cell

Figure 2.3 (Schematic) Opening a gated sodium channel depolarizes the membrane

opens, sodium ions rush in, depolarizing the local membrane and causing the next voltage-gated ion channel to open. The result is a self-propagating wave that travels inexorably down the axon to a synapse. As sodium channels close, the negativity of the inside of that portion of the cell wall increases, *hyperpolarizing* it and inhibiting the propagation of impulses.

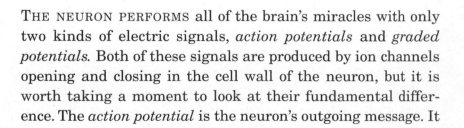

THE NEURON PERFORMS all of the brain's miracles with only two kinds of electric signals, *action potentials* and *graded potentials*. Both of these signals are produced by ion channels opening and closing in the cell wall of the neuron, but it is worth taking a moment to look at their fundamental difference. The *action potential* is the neuron's outgoing message. It is a robust, percussive, staccato signal produced at the point where the axon leaves the cell body. It travels, undiminished, down the full length of the axon to its terminal synapse, where it may signal to other neurons or produce direct behavioral effects in muscles and glands. *Graded potentials* are more subtle and modulated. These tiny charges are the neuron's incoming messages, produced in the dendrites in response to synaptic stimulation. They are also generated in sensory receptors by stimuli such as light, sound, and touch. The neuron listens attentively as the faint signals of graded potentials echo down its many receiving branches toward the cell body, fading as they go. Each one lasts only two-thousandths of a second. However, graded potentials are additive. Their intensity increases in proportion to that of their stimulus—the larger the synaptic stimulation, the greater the dendritic response. A faint chorus of accumulated graded potentials can build to a crescendo and trigger the cymbal crash of an action potential.

Like a bullet, the action potential is an all-or-none response triggered by a specific threshold of excitation. Sometimes called a spike potential, its power is the same whether the trigger is pulled forcefully or weakly, as long as the threshold is exceeded. A stronger stimulus will produce not a larger spike, but more spikes per second. The song of the single neuron can vary from only one spike every few seconds to several hundred spikes per second. It can be sung with any combination of silent intervals and in any rhythm.

The brain produces an infinite variety of music that causes you to laugh, to love, to work, and to wonder how all of this takes place—and it does all of this with only two kinds of electric signals. In 1835, the song of a retinal neuron produced a surprise for early eye surgeons that changed our basic ideas about perception, a reaction that neither they nor their patients were expecting.

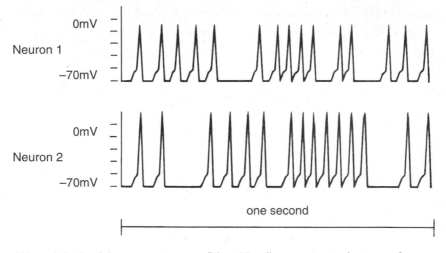

Although both of these neurons are firing 15 spikes per second, neuron 2 sings a different tune than neuron 1, and sings it louder.

Figure 2.4   The songs of two neurons

SURGERY IN THE YEAR 1835 was not for the fainthearted. It would be another decade before William Morton would demonstrate the anesthetic effect of ether. Operations were often performed at home where the patient, the surgeon, and everyone in the neighborhood expected it to be painful and loud. One can imagine how startled ophthalmic surgeons must have been when they first touched the retina with a needle and, instead of pain, their patients experienced distinct flashes of light. In Berlin, Professor Johannes Müller, who is considered by many to be the father of modern physiology, read of this unusual response and immediately recognized its profound implications.

Although philosophers had debated the issue, scientists in 1835 believed that the world exists precisely as it appears, that

51

our senses passively convey the true nature of our surroundings to the mind. Pinpricks producing flashes of light suggested the topsy-turvy notion that the nature of the objects you perceive are determined not by their physical attributes, but by the design of your receptors. Johannes Müller was perhaps the most meticulous, disciplined, and highly respected scientist of the time and was just the man to bring science to bear on this philosophical issue. In the same year that Charles Darwin began exploring the revolutionary implications of the wildlife of the Galápagos Islands, Müller began a thorough investigation of the sense organs. Like Darwin, he came to a radical but cautiously worded conclusion: "Sensation is not the conduction of a quality or state of external bodies to consciousness," but rather, "a conduction of a quality or a state *of our nerves* [italics added] to consciousness, excited by an external cause."[3] In other words, it is you, and not the apple, who determines its redness, aroma, and taste, its shape, color, coolness, texture, and all of the attributes that make it an apple!

The true nature of the "real" world was cast into doubt. In a brave departure from the dogma of centuries, Müller suggested that the world you perceive is a subjective, internal construction determined by the nature of your own nerves. His conclusion is more remarkable when you consider that Müller did not yet know, as we do, that the world and the objects around us are essentially empty space. The atomic particles that swirl about in an apple, table, or chair occupy such a negligible portion of that space, and remain at such astronomical distances from each other relative to their size, that you should be unable to see or feel them. You are aware of those atoms only because of the energy contained in the cloud of electrons that surrounds each of their nuclei. You feel only those atoms whose electrons are able to stimulate your pressure receptors, and you see only those atoms whose electron clouds deflect photons toward your eyes. Even though the atom's nucleus is fifty thousand times more massive than an electron, you have no way to perceive it. You are heedless of that collection of quarks spinning in the atom's center, a mass of particles that, according to some, may be more like vibrating strings wrapped in ten-dimensional "space-time-stuff."[4] The nucleus of the atom is not only difficult to comprehend, it is impossible to perceive.

Out of an obscure block of physical reality, you carve a new one. You create a rich, familiar, perceptual reality out of a strange, physical reality you know very little about. Its interesting features, like those of deep space, are dwarfed by the vastness of the void between them. Energetic clouds of electrons surround imperceptible atomic nuclei like galaxies around a black hole. Photons career about like blazing comets that have no mass and no respect for time or distance. To guide you through a dangerous universe, your mind creates a perceptual reality replete with useful attributes of its own making. From a mysterious mix of forces, particles, and fused dimensions, your sensory neurons select only those properties that matter for the survival of your species. Your mind gives them substance, form, and beauty.

You don't experience a world of whirling electrons buffeting your body and random photons ricocheting into your eyes because your sense organs give your surroundings a complete makeover. The design of your retina, the shape of your ear, the types of receptors in your skin, tongue, and nose create the qualities that you attribute to the familiar world around you. Your sensory receptors produce a specific pattern of brain activity and it is this internal, electric humming that constitutes your very own, homegrown, true-to-life world of people, places, and things.

The world fashioned by the brain is species-specific. Darwin demonstrated that the design of the nervous system is determined by each species' special requirements for survival. Every species will experience the world, its colors and smells, its scope and its scale, uniquely. Each lives in a world that differs from that of every other, and the nature of the "real" world remains a mystery to all. We can dimly guess at the strange world that nourishes the tubeworm in the dark sediment at the crushing depths of the ocean floor. And that world is nothing like the one that fills the heads of sleeping bats as they hang all day from the dark ceiling of a cavern or as they swarm in an amazing display of nocturnal aerobatics using sound waves to catch insects on the wing. Monotonous stretches of open ocean seem to hold endless fascination for gregarious dolphins as they chatter with their pod-mates. And yet, as different as the worlds created by dissimilar brains must be, the basic tools for their construction are shared. Müller taught us to view sensory neurons in a brand-new way. They are not instruments for perceiving our environment. They are the tools that shape it.

The first of these tools to evolve were chemical receptors used by almost every species to define their world with a catalogue of odors, often with thousands more categories than our own. A chemical receptor is nothing more than a tiny depression in a cell wall designed like a lock that only a specific, molecular key will fit. Odor is geometry. You can be strongly attracted to one substance and repelled by another because of only a slight difference in the geometric arrangement of the atoms in their otherwise identical molecules.[5] The most primitive, one-celled organisms drift aimlessly, conserving their energy until the current brings them to a pool of nutrients whose molecular shape fits the locks of their chemical receptors and stimulates purposeful, feeding activity. Scouting ants release a pheromone, a chemical stored in their bodies whose heavy molecules cling to the ground and signal the path toward a food supply to the rest of their colony. Stepping on an ant releases pheromones with much lighter molecules, which dissipate rapidly and signal an alarm for the remaining ants to scatter. Similar locks and keys on the walls of circulating blood cells determine your body's reaction to allergens, viruses, and other invading agents of disease. Along with drifting amoebas, column-forming ants, and skittish, lion-wary antelopes, you have evolved membranes shaped to fit specific chemicals and trigger life-saving responses. When airborne molecular keys fit the locks of your olfactory nerve endings, you will attribute smell to odorless atoms.

Pain and temperature are simply reflections of the speed with which molecules impinge on bare nerve endings, unadorned by any special sensory apparatus. Most of the other tactile nerves in your skin have evolved elaborate sensory endings, which enable you to distinguish between a light breeze through your hair, an insect on your skin, or the impact of a club. The richness of the sense of touch is due to the varied shapes of these nerve endings and their individual sensitivities to different thresholds and vibratory frequencies over areas of different sizes. Each of these tactile receptors responds maximally to an initial touch and to its cessation, but soon ignores a steady pressure—so that you may have to look at your arm to tell if you are still wearing your wristwatch.

Your awareness of your body is aided by proprioceptors, or "self-sensors," which are hidden away within your joints and tendons and respond to their position, stretch, and motion. They provide the feedback needed to compare an activity with its expected result and allow you to reach for a light switch in the dark. These receptors regulate the careful progress of a snail, the stealth of a jaguar, and the grace of a ballerina.

Like the clapper in a bell, a grain of sand is incorporated in the bodies of sea anemones, jellyfish, and corals in such a way as to stimulate sensitive hairs when gravity shifts their position.

This clever signaling arrangement enables the organism to distinguish up from down and to remain upright—and it later evolved into the complex, vestibular apparatus that provides the sense of balance you need to move successfully through the world.

After eons of bumping about in the dark, an early organism gained a distinct advantage by developing a delicate molecule of light-sensitive pigment. Cells containing this pigment were then put to use in several, very different kinds of eyes. One early version arose at the edge of a barnacle shell. This ancient prototype of the eye triggers the crustacean shell to close in response to the passing shadow of a potential predator much as a photoelectric cell operates an automatic door. The octopus developed an eye that is remarkably similar to, although much simpler than, our own, while insects developed eyes from quite another plan. Their honeycomb-shaped, compound eyes trade clarity and fine resolution for an exaggeration of the movements around them. The image of an object moving ever so slightly in space moves completely from one facet of an insect's eye to another, where it suddenly stimulates a brand-new set of receptors. A fly may not recognize who you are, but it is not likely to let you sneak up on it.

The most recently developed sensory apparatus is a group of sensitive hairs that move in response to the vibration of sound waves. The elaborate housing of these delicate nerve endings, protected and yet exposed to minute oscillations of air and water, was the prerequisite for the sophisticated sonar location of bats, whales, and dolphins and, much later, for your hearing, speech, and language.

To say that you have five senses understates and oversimplifies. In addition to smell, taste, touch, sight, and hearing, the five senses recognized by Aristotle, you can sense an increase in the level of carbon dioxide in your blood and respond with increased respiration. Hunger and thirst are your sophisticated responses to your receptors for the acidity, glucose content, and osmotic pressure of your body's fluids, your memory of when you last ate or drank, and the sights, sounds, and smells around you. You are protected against poisons by a special area in your brain stem that, devoid of the protective blood-brain barrier that shields the rest of the brain from unwanted chemicals, responds directly to toxins in your blood and quickly induces nausea and vomiting—an alarm system that at the same time may empty your stomach and save your life.

The brain keeps close tabs on your internal and external environment. It senses the levels of hormones in your blood and regulates their production. When your body is invaded by disease-producing organisms or allergens, it marshals an appropriate immune defense. The endocrine glands and the immune system are now considered to be extended parts of the nervous system. Hormones and white blood cells send messages to the brain and respond to neural signals. The dramatic connection between your physical and mental well-being is rooted in your varied, sensory receptors.

Johannes Müller showed us that your sensory receptors shape your world, but it took rocket science to show us exactly how they do this. The launching of *Sputnik* and the race into outer space provided the tiny tools necessary to discover exactly how the neuron converts environmental changes into the electric impulses of the brain. Micro-engineering produced the first ray of hope that those impulses might be studied in detail.

In spite of their amazing variety, at the heart of every sensory receptor is a transducer, a biological device that transforms energy from the environment into a graded, electric potential. As strange as it seems, touch, sound, and smell produce the same electric result. The biomechanics may vary from one sensory neuron to another, but the electrical outcome is the same. It is only the location and nature of the neurons that

57

respond to those stimuli and the rhythm and timing of their responses that differentiate light from sound, pain from pleasure, fear from amusement, or love from loathing.

However, you will experience none of these sensations unless a signal travels successfully across a *synapse*. Signals do not pass through the brain like electricity through a collection of copper wires. It is the exquisite selectivity of the synapse that accounts for discrete perceptions rather than sensory static, for coordinated movements rather than frenetic seizures, for intellect rather than brutishness; and this ingenious communication center linking one neuron with another is where we are "turned on and turned off."

The term synapse refers to the specialized, *presynaptic membrane* at the end of an axon, the *postsynaptic membrane* on the dendrite of its neighboring neuron, and the *synaptic cleft* between them, a space measuring about 25 nanometers— or 25-millionths of a millimeter across.

When an action potential arrives at the end of its axon, it causes a calcium-ion–gated channel to briefly open. A sudden influx of calcium releases stored chemical transmitter molecules to float across the synaptic cleft like grains of pollen from a blossom. The postsynaptic membrane of the neuron at the opposite shore has a collection of very sophisticated chemical receptors. Only if a transmitter molecule is precisely shaped to fit into one of these receptor molecules, will it become embedded and trigger a response. Here, in the dendrite of the receiving neuron, the miracle of recognition occurs. One neuron acknowledges another and a new, graded potential is generated—*but only if the proper conditions are met*. The situation reminds me of a cartoon I once saw showing a blackboard completely filled with a string of mathematical notations and a professor who says, "This still needs a little work right here."

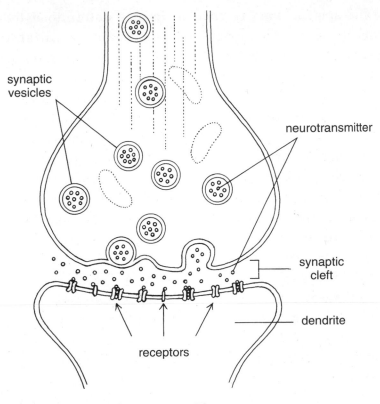

synaptic
vesicles

neurotransmitter

synaptic
cleft

dendrite

receptors

Figure 2.5   The synapse

He is pointing to a notation scribbled in brackets halfway through the equation: "[Here, a miracle occurs]."

As your brain appears to sit there doing nothing, gated ion channels are fluttering like key stops on a clarinet, regulating the flow of charged particles in and out of every neuron. The electric notes they produce ripple down the cell membrane and, as each note reaches a synapse, its energy opens a gate for calcium ions. The influx of calcium bursts a pod of vesicles whose molecules carry a signal across the synapse to a neighboring neuron and encourage it to sing in turn.

The specific song of each neuron is determined by the signals it hears, and it listens to a very complex musical score. One neuron may have many thousands of synapses and a chorus of thousands of graded potentials can travel down its dendrites toward its cell body. Here, the neruon reads the score and immediately composes a melodic response. In a matter of milliseconds, it dispatches a brand-new set of notes down its axon toward another set of synapses for its neighbors to hear. The neuron is essentially a monotone in terms of the amplitude and shape of its signals as they appear on an oscilloscope. The notes of one neuron may differ from those of another, but each neuron can sing only one. And yet, by producing its note with varying rhythms, timing, and frequency, each neuron can produce a limitless repertoire. It can sing a monotone version of "The Flight of the Bumblebee" or "The Tennessee Waltz."

But not every signal arriving at a synapse is passed across. Modulating brain chemicals, *neuromodulators* such as dopamine and serotonin can act as border agents, blocking some signals and enhancing others to influence your moods, thoughts, and behavior. In sharp contrast with ordinary neurotransmitters that act in milliseconds, the influence of neuromodulators is slow in onset and can last for minutes, hours, days, or even longer.[6,7] At every moment, whether with a trumpet blast or with a precisely timed silence, each neuron contributes to the electric symphony that is your current state of mind. The taste of a peach, the view from your window, the next choice you make or action you take, each of these is a composition of signals from the entire membership of your one-of-a-kind orchestra of neurons. It is an electric melody, modulated by chemistry. However, you will not hear any of this music by holding your ear to someone's skull. It is just loud enough to be heard a few millionths of a millimeter away from its source.

THE ELECTROCHEMICAL MUSIC of the brain was first recorded in 1929 by a German psychiatrist, Dr. Hans Berger. Connecting an electrode on his scalp to an amplifier, he converted electrical impulses from the brain into the movement of a pen oscillating over a sheet of paper in rapid, medium-amplitude waves, which he named *alpha* waves. His report received little attention until the 1940s, when it was found that rhythmic alpha waves become markedly erratic during an epileptic seizure. Curiosity about possible clinical applications of Berger's "brain waves" led to the development of more sophisticated electroencephalogram (EEG) machines with multiple electrodes recording simultaneously from several areas on the scalp. Although little could be told about their exact source or their meaning, abnormal brain waves were soon noted in many other conditions, including brain tumors, encephalitis, and stroke. In addition to alpha waves, much larger and slower *delta* waves were recorded during sleep, and extremely small, rapid *theta* waves were recorded during stress. By the 1950s the wavy lines produced by these recordings and the observation of periodic, rapid eye movements in sleeping infants showed us that your noisy chorus of neurons gives regularly scheduled performances, even as you sleep.

It was long believed that sleep was boring, that reducing your sensory stimulation and resting your muscles was simply matched with a diminished activity of the brain. The EEG proved the contrary. During sleep, the brain behaves as though it is entering a gym where it performs repetitive workouts lasting approximately ninety minutes each. These periodic performances have been given the name rapid-eye-movement (REM) cycles because of the ocular activity that accompanies them. During REM sleep, the brain is actively involved in the creation of dream imagery and the eyes seem to follow the imagined action with movements that can be short and darting or wide and sweeping, just as when you look around with your eyes open. Intense electrical activity can be recorded from the retina and from the portions of the brain involved with vision. During REM sleep, EEG waves everywhere have a normal alpha rhythm, just as small and fast as when you are awake, but recordings of the electrical activity from your major muscle groups is reduced to zero. While you dream, the body is plunged into its deepest state of paralysis, thus protecting you from "sleepwalking."

Energetic REM cycles are followed by quiet intermissions, cycles of deep sleep, during which EEG tracings show larger, slower delta waves. There is no movement of the eyes and no electrical activity coming from them; however, the electrical activity coming from the major muscle groups is almost as great as when you are awake. Paradoxically, tossing and turning are common during the cycles of your deepest sleep.

Two recent reports demonstrate an imaginative and unexpectedly valuable application of Berger's curious brain waves. These relate to the often ballyhooed concept of biofeedback. Originally greeted with appropriate skepticism, this idea has gradually gained respect. There have been many demonstrations that, with an appropriate investment of time and training, you can produce limited but measurable effects on your brain waves, your blood pressure, and other functions usually considered involuntary. Two remarkable examples were published in 1999. The first was a report of three patients who were taught to use the brain waves recorded by an EEG to control their artificial limbs. Electrodes from the scalp were connected to the cursor control on a computer screen, which in turn controlled the patient's prosthetic hand. In each case, after six months of training, the patient was able to use the EEG signal to direct his prosthesis to pick up a weight, use a fork, and lift a cup.[8]

A second report requires a brief prologue in order to appreciate its impact. Imagine being paralyzed to the point of being unable to move a single muscle in your body, not even to lift a finger or to make a sound. This is a reality for a small number of people who exist in this nightmarish, "locked-in" state with absolutely no means of communication, an active mind trapped in the body of a vegetable. A team of American and European researchers, led by Dr. Niels Birbaumer of the University of Tübingen in Germany, had two such patients undergo training, similar to that in the prosthetic hand study, lasting hundreds of sessions until they were able to achieve 75 percent effectiveness in creating "spikes" of EEG brain activity on demand. These spikes were used as signals to select individual letters of the alphabet displayed on a computer screen and to laboriously construct words and sentences, typically at a rate of only two or three characters per minute. The first message ever constructed in this manner was a twelve-line thank-you note to the researchers. That message took its grateful author sixteen hours to compose, but the joy and relief that it conveyed could be expressed in no other way.[9]

EEG recordings from the scalp provide only rather general information about the song of the neuron, a bit like the sounds of a noisy party heard from an apartment across the hall. The level and character of those sounds might convey a rough idea of what is going on, but reveal nothing about the individual conversations accompanying the hors d'oeuvres. That level of detail would require recordings from individual neurons. The interest and ability to record the signals of individual neurons arose in the early 1950s, and we have been improving our ability to decode those messages ever since. Recording instruments capture the frequency, rhythm, amplitude, and timing of neural signals, but we may have not yet even guessed at the most important features of that code. Only during the 1990s, the period that President Bush designated the Decade of the Brain, did we begin to recognize the subtlety and richness that account for the wealth of information conveyed by each neuron. That signal is now being analyzed at an unprecedented level of detail and, at long last, the particulars of the electrical events upon which your behavior and survival depend are finally coming vaguely into view.

Within the last few years, a most remarkable recording technique has been developed. Using the same techniques used to fabricate printed circuits and computer chips, technicians in specially designed "clean rooms," wearing surgical garb and working at glass-hooded, ventilated benches, are crafting computer chips that can simultaneously analyze signals from large numbers of selected neurons as well as from several sites in a single cell, in awake subjects. Because these listening posts can be arranged flexibly in three dimensions, it is possible to tell which messages are going where, which come from a single neuron, and which come from many, whether they occur simultaneously or in tandem, whether they respond to each other or go on independently. The collected data is being stored in computers and analyzed in that ultimate language of the universe—mathematics. For the first time, we are getting direct, high-fidelity, stereophonic, live recordings of the choral music of one hundred billion neurons and we are beginning to learn their lyrics.

Whether you are asleep or awake, each neuron continuously modulates its rhythm and tempo. As though following the baton of a conductor, it responds to changes in your attention, periods of light and dark, and changes in the concentration of modulating chemicals. While responding to these important cues, each neuron continues to produce its unique and highly interpretive notes. No two neurons sound exactly alike. Like a Stradivarius violin, the nature of its response depends not only

64

on the musical score that it reads from its dendrites, but on its distinctive shape and timbre honed during the evolutionary development of that particular cell—qualities imbued by its DNA. Its melody is shaped by the precise number and location of its synapses, the structure of its synaptic membranes, and the nature of the chemical messengers within them. The neuron also learns as it plays. In Chapter 8 you will see how its music is shaped not only by evolution's mold, but by the indelible stamp of experience. Your individuality springs from its expanding repertoire. Within the complexity of the neuron, we have discovered an intelligence that is the source of our own.

On the weekend of March 22–23, 1996, a workshop was held in the Laboratory of Cognitive Neurobiology at Boston University. The purpose was to discuss the revolutionary new method of recording not just from one neuron, but from large numbers of them. This evolving technology of multichannel, microelectrode data collection and analysis, then in use for only a few years, was already amassing huge databases from which a new level of understanding the music of the neuron is possible. The organizers of that conference, Joel L. Davis of the Office of Naval Research and Howard Eichenbaum of Boston University, published a review of the rapidly expanding body of literature regarding this new field of research. Using language that is unusually strong for a scientific work, they suggest that decoding these recordings "will bring about a revolution in our conceptions about the brain and test our most radical hypotheses about the emergent properties of neural interaction."[10]

The emergent properties that they allude to are nothing less than the subjective products of the brain such as seeing, imagining, and remembering. The inescapable conclusion is that the massive data being collected in these recordings will test our conjectures and theories about how we *experience* life. Neuroscience is finally bringing consciousness into the laboratory.

3

The Ghost in the Machine

The Elusive Homunculus

NEUROSCIENTISTS USE the shorthand term *the hard problem* to describe the struggle to understand consciousness, awareness, free will, and the biological basis of our sense of self. Until 1990, this area was not even considered to be a legitimate subject of scientific inquiry. That changed during the Decade of the Brain, as technology dramatically narrowed the gap between theoretical and experimental brain science. Although the hard problem remains an elusive target, it is being approached with new techniques and with renewed vigor. A fascinating compilation of research papers devoted solely to this subject is published monthly in the *Journal of Consciousness Studies*. Among the editors of this journal are such prominent cognitive scientists as Bernard Baars and Daniel Dennett; philosophers David Chalmers and John Searle; psychologists Benjamin Libet and Walter Freeman; as well as distinguished psychiatrists, psychologists, physicists, mathematicians, religious leaders, and sociologists from the world's leading academic institutions. This pursuit still raises a few incredulous eyebrows. However, the undulating, relentlessly rising tide of scientific insight has repeatedly washed away the footprints of skeptics who, as they watched from the shore, declared at every stage that *this* was as far as it would go.

Our current high-water mark, the question now at the leading edge of neuroscience, is defined by the old riddle of whether a tree falling out of earshot makes any noise. What is the real stuff of conscious experience? What is the physical and biological nature of *qualia* (a word coined by neuroscientists to describe subjective experiences such as sight and sound)? What *exactly* is insight?

A tree crashing to the forest floor certainly sets up sound waves that can be measured by inanimate instruments, and it creates electrical patterns of activity in the brain that correlate with the sound of a falling tree. But that does not explain the mystery. We are left with a magic trick. A facsimile of the tree and the forest is fabricated in your head. Inaudible signals traveling through your inner-space galaxy of neurons produce an alarming, unexpected noise in a virtual universe—all within your brain. If neither you nor anyone else is there to hear it, the falling tree stirs up dust and sound waves, but it makes no such noise. The objective events of colliding masses and vibrating air waves are not sufficient to do that job. Even the addition of neural excitation is not enough. The subjective phenomena of human experience depend on something else. Identifying and understanding that something else, explaining the experience of consciousness, is the ultimate, vexing challenge for neuroscience. There are now almost as many theories of consciousness as there are theorists and experimental researchers studying this question.

When Wilder Penfield and his co-workers outlined areas on the cortex that correspond to every part of the body, the resulting cartoonlike tracings conjured up the age-old idea of a homunculus, a little man within the brain. It certainly feels as if there is a central, magical place inside your head toward which all sensory information flows and from which all behaviors emanate. There, it seems that someone or something—a ghost in the machine—interprets your sensations and authors your response. Galen and Descartes each had their own choice for the single place from which a ghostly spirit controls the body.

Today, we are faced with an embarrassment of riches. We have found dozens of areas scattered throughout your brain that interpret sensations and initiate behavior. The ghost in the machine has become a family of goblins and each appears to inhabit a discrete location. We have assigned them to cramped compartments and have ascribed an unreasonable degree of autonomy to each one. We attach exaggerated significance to the functional segregation within the brain's lumpy anatomy, and a misguided hyperbole has crept into our vocabulary. We say that one area of the brain "processes" vision and another "produces" hearing; that one bump in the cortex "controls" speech while another one "moves" your arm. The right brain has been credited with your talent for music, the left with your mathematical ability, and we have begun to speak of "right-brained" and "left-brained" people. If there is a ghost in the machine, a spirit or a soul, it is moving gleefully about playing hide-and-seek and giving us a tantalizingly incomplete view of its nature and its location.

Speculating on the available evidence, most neuroscientists have given up the ghost. They have abandoned the idea that a separate soul inhabits your flesh and bones. The preponderance of evidence suggests that you are reducible to neural activity and that your behavior is determined by natural events. The best bet is that the qualia, the mysterious phenomena of subjective experience, consciousness, and free will, arise solely from the enormous complexity of the neurons and the intricacies of their minute signals. The majority opinion holds that the miracle of subjective experience is an *emergent property* of your brain. However, you might get differing definitions of the term emergent property from biologists, psychologists, philosophers, theologians, chaos theorists, particle physicists, and all of the others who now contribute freely and sometimes passionately to this area of neuroscience.

There is no question that the area of the brain that contributes to your sense of self more than any other is the frontal lobe, in particular, that part of the frontal cortex that is situated forward of the area that was demonstrated by Penfield to contribute to voluntary movements. There is compelling, new evidence that the *prefrontal cortex,* making use of information coming from every other part of your brain, builds your sense of self from scratch.

In the days when electroshock treatment and frontal lobotomy were among the few available therapies for certain behavioral disorders, these had an almost immediate effect. Stunning the prefrontal cortex with seizure-inducing jolts of electricity or severing its connections to the rest of the brain alleviated depression and psychotic ideation; however, these procedures also severely diminished the patient's working memory, ability to plan, capacity to theorize about other people's minds, and ability to feel empathy. Treated patients were simply no longer themselves and, given the alternative, that was considered an improvement. The frontal lobe was recognized even then as having a great deal to do with your sense of who you really are.

In October 1999, Dr. Elizabeth Gould and Dr. Charles Gross of Princeton University showed us *how* we build a sense of self.[1] Theirs was one of those discoveries that force us to abandon deeply entrenched beliefs. The long-accepted dictum that adults never generate new brain cells is headed for the trash heap. Gould and Cross found that thousands of fresh, newly born neurons arrive at the frontal cortex each day. The source of this daily delivery is the sheet of ependymal cells that line the brain's ventricles. This layer of cells has long been known to produce neurons in the embryo, but it is now recognized that it continues to turn out new neurons throughout life. Galen may not have been that far off. It is not fluid in the ventricles, but the cellular lining of their walls, that is responsible for our vitality. Even more startling was Gould's and Gross's finding that, as each fresh batch of neurons arrives at the frontal cortex in conveyor-belt fashion, those new cells form interconnecting synapses with one another and act as a cohesive unit. They record a day's worth of perceptions from the rest of the brain and establish a date-tagged file of memories. Memories engraved in the circuitry of the cerebral cortex, growing by the day, are the stuff your self is made of. The California Institute of Technology's theoretical neuroscientist, Steven Quartz, put it nicely: "The key to building a human being lies in letting the world help build the prefrontal cortex as the prefrontal cortex experiences the world."[2]

But something is missing. If you are nothing but a collection of perceptions and memories magically stored in the neural activity of your brain, how can you surprise us with something unexpected, something not determined by prior events? Where in this model is there room for your free will? The answer from most neuroscientists who have studied this question is not one you will like to hear. They will tell you that there is none. There is no "you" in there calling the shots, no ghost in the machine directing behavior, just the machine itself, generating incredible, electrical patterns that record perceptions, process behavior, imitate, replicate, and learn. Ultimately, your brain is just reacting. It creates only the *illusion* of self-direction.

This most unsettling view gained surprising credence from

a famous experiment by the University of California at San Francisco neurophysiologist Benjamin Libet in 1985.[3] The design of the study is simple, but explaining the results is not. His subjects were asked to watch a spot revolving on a clock face in front of them and, at a time of their choosing, to flex their wrists. They were told to note exactly where the spot was when they decided to act. With strategically placed recording electrodes, Libet measured two things: *the time the action began* and a brain wave called *the readiness potential,* an electrical pattern seen just before any complex action takes place. Invariably, the readiness potential occurred *before,* not after, the moment of their "decision." The brain begins its activity *before* you "decide" that you want it to. If the readiness potential occurs before your "intention," you are deluding yourself with your notion of free will. A shocking and depressing conclusion.

However, Libet's experiment holds out a modest hope that we do exercise some control of our lives, that we do make free choices. Although the "decision" to act came *after* the readiness potential, it still came *before* the action. There is a fraction of a second during which one could theoretically decide *not* to take the action the brain has prepared. You *can* just say no. Volition may consist merely of stifling inappropriate urges. We have to wait patiently for ideas to come along but, if we don't like them, we can exercise immediate veto power as they bubble to the surface. If we do not exercise our veto during that brief window of opportunity, we will delude ourselves into believing that we initiated that idea or action from its inception. We will believe that we authored the bill rather than that we simply passed up the chance to kill it. However, we have to stay on our toes. We have only about two-tenths of a second in which to say no—and we get no second chances. Perhaps it is this degree of vigilance that wears us out by the end of the day and produces our need for sleep. And then, after we have fallen asleep at the switch, a wild assortment of ideas bubbles uncensored into our dreams.

Even with this loophole, with this idea of a *free won't* rather than a free will, it is difficult to accept that our ability to initiate an action, our capacity to surprise, is nothing but an illusion. The brain would have to be extremely good at deception to trick us into believing that an involuntary reaction is something that we actively willed. And as it turns out, there is a wealth of clinical evidence that the brain does indeed deceive us. Oliver Sacks has chronicled several amusing and poignant cases of this in *The Man Who Mistook His Wife for a Hat, and Other Clinical Tales* (Touchstone Books, 1998).

Brain lesions involving the right cerebral cortex cause some patients to find nothing unusual about wearing their coat with only one arm through a sleeve, and they concoct elaborate explanations for doing so, bizarre stories that suit them just fine. They maintain the delusion that the left half of their body simply does not belong to them. They have no recognition of its obvious absurdity even though it subjects them to real danger when, for example, they sit down for a bath while the left side of their body remains outside the tub. Drugs, disease, and the delirium tremens of an alcoholic going suddenly dry can produce hallucinations and delusions, deceptions that are frighteningly real.

It may be that creating illusions is what the normal brain does for a living. The uncomfortable view is emerging that your sense of self and your belief in the voluntary nature of your actions are fabrications—illusions useful for survival, embroidered by an inherited set of neurons reacting to your perceptions and memories—designed to put the best face on things and to get you through the day the best they can. It appears that there is no one inside your head watching what goes on and deciding what to do. There is only the brain, every part of it watching every other, a house of mirrors.

It is more than mildly disturbing to think of free will as an illusion. You build your reputation on the choices you make, and you expect others to take responsibility for theirs. Francis Crick has resurrected your personal accountability by stating this disconcerting view of volition in another, perhaps more palatable way,[4] which I have distilled as follows: You might be aware of making several plans for a future action and of a decision to act on one of them. However, you are not conscious of everything that goes on in the brain. Most of the intricate computations that led to that decision (I assume he would include here your ambitions, desire for approval, fears, resentments, jealousies, and memories of similar experiences and their consequences) are unavailable for immediate recall. Like much of the brain's activity, the convoluted decision-making process that produces your behavior goes on in microseconds and is largely unknown to you. You did choose and act, carefully weighing in an instant the interests of your emotions and intellect. But you know that only after the fact.

This view, that your behavior is determined by predictable (though complex and often obscure) events, is not unanimous. There are some high-powered proponents of Descartes's dualism still separating mind from body and still betting that somewhere in the brain we will find what Daniel Dennett, with tongue in cheek, calls the Cartesian Theater.[5] They believe that there is a place or perhaps several places in the brain that in some way, not reducible to matter and not determined by previous events, perform the mystical function that Descartes once attributed to heavenly spirits acting through the pineal gland. An active search continues for some force, spirit or soul, a ghost in the machine capable of breaking free of the bonds

73

of determinism, capable of unpredictable behavior and free choice. It is something we intuitively feel within us and would be gratified to find.

The most notable proponent of a soul hidden somewhere in the brain is the Nobel Prize–winning neurophysiologist Sir John Eccles, who suspects that the mystery of consciousness and the strangeness of the quantum world may be interconnected. Common to them both is the principle of uncertainty. Physicists have determined that it is impossible to know with certainty both the position and the velocity of an electron, and this principle of quantum mechanics, the uncertainty principle, allows for unpredictable events. Substituting probability for certainty affords a refuge from rigid determinism.[6,7] The mathematician Roger Penrose has postulated that consciousness arises from certain quantum mechanical activity within the neuron and he has even proposed the precise structure within the neuron, the microtubule, where this consciousness-producing process occurs.[8] Gerald Edelman, a molecular biologist and writer with a special interest in neuroscience, believes that consciousness and spontaneity reside in a complex arrangement of circular circuits in the brain. His descriptions of "reentrant loops" responsible for the miracle of self-awareness and free will have left even many brain scientists going around in circles.[9] Michael Gazzaniga, a pioneer in the study of the differences between the right and left halves of the brain and the Director of the Center for Cognitive Neuroscience at Dartmouth College, points to evidence of a biological "interpreter" located in the left hemisphere.[10] The competing theories of consciousness are complex and the latest views of their leading proponents can be reviewed at leisure in the *Journal of Conscious Studies.*[11]

The exciting truth is that we no longer need to idly speculate as to whether—or where—a ghost might lurk in the machine, and we can finally move beyond our fascination with isolated lobes and fissures. The answers will be found in the flood of information now pouring in from the laboratories of neuro-physiologists, molecular biologists, and the human genome project. It may take years to decipher the huge wave of information that is currently being generated, but the tide is rising and the surf is up; this is hardly the time for stodgy pessimism. To better understand my unabashed optimism, it will help to know more about the research that fosters it, much of which has centered on vision.

4

The Photon and Your Brain

Your Quiet Conversation with Nature

IT IS LITTLE WONDER THAT the story of Genesis begins with light. This welcome, radiant energy is responsible not only for vision, but also for photosynthesis of the nutrients that sustain us. The miracle of vision and the staff of life are both children of the photon, the unimaginably tiny packet of energy that illuminates the world around you. The photon is central to this story because it also lights up the world within your brain.

When you ponder your ability to see, you probably shake your head slightly and dismiss it as a miracle. For most of us, in spite of widely available information to the contrary, it still seems as though the eyes capture an image of the outside world and send it fully formed for the mystical mind to appreciate. Vision is truly a chain of miracles. It begins in a lamp filament above your chair or in the furious heat of a distant star, where unseen atoms change their energy level and release photons. Escaping from a mysterious world of electrons and quarks, these parcels of pure energy go from 0 to 670 million miles per hour in no time flat. Photons hurtle through space as fast as anything in this universe can travel, and then bounce silently off this page. Some of them strike the visual pigment at the back of your eyes where, like fingers landing on piano keys, they come to an attention-grabbing stop. After dazzling you with the announcement of their arrival, they disappear once again into the quantum world from which they came. During the next fraction of a second, in the total darkness of your skull, networks of neurons construct a facsimile of this page—as well as an echo of my thoughts as I wrote these words. Perhaps it is equally miraculous that we have come to understand how that happens.

At the beginning of the twentieth century, physicists were struggling to understand the mystery of light, anatomists were beginning to contemplate the secrets of the neuron—and neither group suspected how the pieces of their two puzzles would intertwine.

BY THE TIME ANATOMISTS discovered the neuron, physics was very nearly a dead science. Sir Isaac Newton had long ago defined the fundamental laws of nature and physicists had exhausted themselves devising new ways to test their validity. If you dropped weights from the Tower of Pisa, started a pendulum swinging, or struck a taut piano string, as long as you took careful measurements, you knew exactly what to expect. The Newtonian universe was an exquisitely made grandfather clock, wound and running according to plan.

Light, however, remained a pesky problem. As it speeds from its source to its destination, light blithely defies Newton's well-respected laws. It was known in 1900 that light is part of the electromagnetic spectrum of radiant energy described by James Maxwell, and that it behaves like waves traveling across a pond. But light posed two riddles whose answers would revitalize physics, give us a new understanding of the universe, and teach us how we interact with our environment.

First, unlike sound and other waves that require a medium to convey them, light waves can pass through a vacuum. For a while, this led to the mistaken belief that there is a mysterious substance that propagates light and, undetected, fills a vacuum as well as all of the otherwise empty space in the universe. Physicists named this theoretical medium the *ether* and devised experiments to measure the speed of light traveling through it. This raised a second mystery having to do with relativity. A ball thrown toward you from the front of a train would travel more quickly if the train were traveling toward you, and it would take much longer to reach you if the train were speeding backward. The speed of light, however, was found to be constant, whether coming from the headlamp of an approaching locomotive, from one speeding backward or from another standing at the station. Light, alone in nature, was immune to Newton's law of relative motion.

In 1902, denied the teaching position he had hoped for, an undistinguished but fiercely curious graduate of Switzerland's Federal Institute of Technology accepted an unassuming position as a patent inspector in Bern. There, he devoted his abundant spare time to studying light's refusal to obey the law. After years of wrestling with the problem, one afternoon while on a walk in the mountains he suddenly came to an astonishing conclusion, one that defies logic. Since speed is simply the distance traveled in a unit of time, the only way to explain this pesky, constant speed of light was to conclude that time and distance vary with speed!

In 1905, Albert Einstein published a theory so provocative, yet so elegant, that it brought the leading physicists of the world to the Bern patent office to meet its obscure, young author. His

Special Theory of Relativity challenged Newton's and nearly every one else's assumption that time and distance are absolute. Einstein declared that for a man on a moving train, the minute is longer and the mile is shorter than for his friend at the station. He proposed that as one approaches the speed of light, distances grow smaller and time slows down. He described the speed of light as a universal speed limit at which distances shrink to zero and time stands still. The study of light produced disquieting cracks in the rigid structure of Newtonian physics.

The cracks grew wider as it appeared that light behaves not only like waves traveling at the universal speed limit, but like particles as well. In his subsequent work, *The General Theory of Relativity,* Einstein suggested that, like particles and planets, light needs no help from an imaginary ether to travel across a vacuum, and that gravity will pull light into a curving trajectory as it passes near a star. In 1919, a group of British scientists sailed to the South Atlantic to observe a solar eclipse and to test this radical hypothesis. If true, the light coming from a star known to be behind the sun would be pulled by the sun's gravity into a curving path and would be visible to them. The star would appear next to the eclipsed sun, where they knew it was not! This prospect quickly captured the imagination of the general public. When the star appeared exactly as his *General Theory of Relativity* had predicted, the news appeared in banner headlines around the world and the British experiment in the South Seas became the subject of a popular, silent film. Albert Einstein became a household topic of conversation in a world eager to talk about something other than the horrific years of war that had just ended.

In those heady, postwar years, a new physics was born that proclaimed that the world is not as it seems. We were left to grapple with space and time, which not only vary with speed, but are fused and curved as well. We find ourselves in a universe where mass and energy are interchangeable, comprised of basic elements that behave sometimes like waves, sometimes like particles and always unpredictably. Almost as an afterthought, Einstein calculated that every bit of matter contains as much energy as its mass multiplied by the enormous speed of light—squared! This now famous relationship, $E = mc^2$, was verified decades later, at Los Alamos, Hiroshima, and Nagasaki, and led to banner headlines of a different sort at the end of another world war. Albert Einstein's sudden revelation along a mountain trail permanently changed our view of the universe in ways he could not have suspected. It also set the stage for understanding vision.

The study of light as it travels through time and space has always had a profound and unexpected influence on our view of nature. The Greeks found a harmony in the orderly rotation of the stars, which they described as the music of the spheres. For centuries, church ceilings echoed with open tones and harmonies inspired by images of that celestial order. When Sir Isaac Newton described fixed, predictable laws of the universe, the meandering, open-ended Gregorian chant was replaced by the precision of the metronome and the rules of measure and key. In the early twentieth century, when a star appeared where it should not have been, musical notes began to appear where they were not expected in the syncopation of ragtime and jazz. Our bizarre, new understanding of light, time, and space began to appear in the paintings of cubists, abstract expressionists, and surrealists. Today, perceptions that were once the province of theoretical physicists and misunderstood artists are shared generally. Our expanding experience continues to shape our view of the universe.

Accumulated experience also molds the individual brain. In Chapter 8 you will see unmistakable evidence that sensory input is the food necessary to build the brain's connections.

Studying the neurology of vision taught us that experience physically changes the brain, and that discovery has fundamentally changed our understanding of how the environment shapes our lives. Learning how visual image is constructed sheds light on the brain's development as well as its function, on the fascinating life of the neuron as well as your own. This construction project begins in the *photoreceptors*, light-sensitive neurons that interact directly with that fleet fugitive from the atoms of distant stars, the photon.

Much of what we know about the brain we learned from studying the retina, a thin sheet of neurons at the back of the eye. An outgrowth of the brain, the retina is evolution's satellite dish for the photon. When your embryo was less than one quarter of an inch long, about the size of a large grain of rice, and well before you acquired any of the features that later would mark you as human, your fetal brain developed two bulges where young neurons would acquire the amazing capacity to recognize the photon and signal its arrival. At this point, your brain was just a slight enlargement at the front end of a hollow tube. Later, that tube would differentiate into your *central nervous system,* your brain, spinal cord, motor and sensory peripheral nerves; as well as your *autonomic nervous system,* the group of nerves regulating your automatic bodily functions.

The powerful, persistent, evolutionary influence of the photon caused two areas of your developing brain tissue to elongate and stretch toward a location where reception would be better, toward the surface of your tadpolelike, embryonic face. Upon their arrival at this new location, these budding neurons initiated the construction of your window to the world, and our window to the brain.

Photons have rained on Earth since its beginning, pelting it with a bombardment that cannot be felt, smelled, tasted, or heard. Primitive organisms, previously concerned only with

forebrain

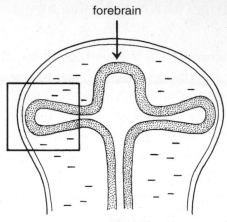

4 mm embryo

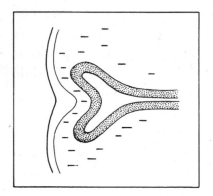

5 mm embryo

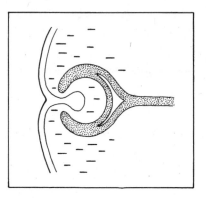

8 mm embryo

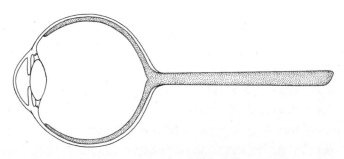

Figure 4.1 Your retina is an outgrowth of your brain

internal or very local matters, eventually developed a small area sensitive to these peculiar, telecommunicating packets of light. As this new "photon detector" evolved, it played a key role in defining for each species its particular place in the universe. At dawn's dim signal, earthworms return to the safety of the dark, moist soil. Honeybees are guided by beacons of polarized light, invisible to us, which punctuate their nearly colorless world and lead them to the nectar-laden centers of dull, gray flowers. From an eagle's mountain perch, the magnified image of a tiny movement on the valley floor triggers a ferocious dive.

Of our five senses, sight alone extends human awareness to the stars and has led to momentous conclusions about our place among them. With a crude telescope, Galileo saw tiny moons orbiting Jupiter and confirmed the humbling notion that we do not stand at the center of the universe. Edwin Hubble recognized a peculiar, red shift in the color of starlight as a measure of the speed at which the universe has been expanding since its explosive birth. We have analyzed the gasses of exploding stars and found the stuff of which we are made. And all of this hinged on the peculiar shape of a single, remarkable molecule, *the visual pigment.*

In 1967, Dr. George Wald was awarded a Nobel Prize for deciphering the beginning of what he called "our quiet conversation with Nature."[1] He had discovered how a delicate molecule of purple pigment, coiled like a tiny, spring-loaded door chime hidden inside the photoreceptor cell, announces the arrival of the photon and transforms its energy into a neural impulse that your brain can understand.

To truly appreciate light perception is to understand what an unlikely event it is. A harsh reality is trivialized by the bland statement that visible light is a "small part" of the total spectrum of electromagnetic energy radiating from the sun and stars. That "small part" is the number one preceded by fourteen zeros and a decimal point, one million times smaller than the parts per billion used to measure trace elements in drinking water.

If the wavelengths of the total spectrum of energy radiating to Earth were represented on a strip of paper stretched across the United States, visible light would take up only two millionths of an inch of that list somewhere in Nebraska. Extending westward would be a list of invisible X rays with their high energy and shorter wavelength. The roster reaching from the plains to the East Coast would denote invisible heat and radio waves of lower energy and longer wavelength. Only that microscopic section near Omaha would register the photons with just the right energy and wavelength to react with the pigment in your retina, visible light. Not only are we dependent on this minuscule part of the electromagnetic spectrum, the rest is lethal.

Space suits protect against more than just extremes of temperature, they shield against X rays and microwaves that would kill instantly. Ultraviolet light waves shorter than 300 millimicrons denature proteins, break apart nucleic acids, and prevent normal cell development. Wavelengths longer than 2,000 millimicrons are too "hot" for sustained life. Fortunately, our atmosphere absorbs most of the radiation above and below those critical limits and it most readily admits those photons with wavelengths near 500 millimicrons. This wavelength is compatible with life, it is utilized by plants in photosynthesis, it is very near the center of the visible spectrum, and it paints our sunlit sky a glorious blue. Our amiable atmosphere selectively admits that one *quadrillionth* of the total spectrum of radiant energy that warms and lights our world. Visible light is a magical blend of contradictions, insubstantial and yet vital, obscure and yet revealing, abundant and yet surprisingly rare.

To see and *to look* are active verbs. Until the seventeenth century, most people regarded vision as an active process, the result of a vital energy that, when you will it to do so, exits the eye from a mysterious, internal source. It even seemed that you could regulate this force voluntarily, making glances either hard or soft, threatening or beguiling, warm or cold. The potential force of this "visual spirit" was felt to be so great that ancient Egyptians painted the symbol of Horus, the god of light, on their homes to protect against the "evil eye." I can remember my parents often saying "keine hora" upon hearing good news, a Yiddish expression meant as a wish that your good fortune should escape the attention of that evil spirit.

In fact, vision does require some of your energy, but this energy is expended before, not during the act of seeing. Much like the energy required to wind a spring, metabolic energy is continuously expended to assemble and then reassemble an extraordinary molecule of purple pigment in every photoreceptor cell in your retina.

Two things set your visual pigment molecule apart from any other pigment found in nature. First, it defines for you what is visible light by absorbing only those electromagnetic waves measuring between 380 and 760 millimicrons (.00038 and .00076 millimeters) from the crest of one wave to the crest of the next. You do not see ultraviolet or infrared light simply because this finicky molecule does not absorb their wavelengths. Second, the visual pigment molecule is so delicately constructed that, like a house of cards, the energy of even a single photon breaks it apart and triggers the electrical event that allows you to see. Each of your 250 million photoreceptor cells continuously builds and stores about 100 million molecules of visual pigment.

There are about 125 million rods and cones—photoreceptor cells named for their shape—in each of your eyes. The smaller rods respond to dim light and allow for your limited night vision. The fatter cones respond to bright light and come in three flavors, with visual pigments that maximally absorb light with either shorter (blue) wavelengths, medium (green) wavelengths, or longer (red) wavelengths, providing the basis for color discrimination. The dense concentration of cones at the center of the retina permits the resolution of fine details such as the letters on this page.

The spectacular phenomenon of vision hinges, quite literally, on a minute detail. George Wald discovered that the door chime rung by an arriving photon is nothing more than a chain of carbon atoms in a molecule of vitamin A. Normally these atoms are arranged in a straight row like an arm fully extended. In the rare form of vitamin A that is incorporated in your visual pigment, that carbon chain is bent at the elbow. The added energy gained from absorbing even a single photon springs it straight. That tiny bit of energy strengthens the bond between two carbon atoms at the bend in the chain just enough to snap them back into a straight line. This is the hair trigger that sets off the miracle of vision.

Once its carbon chain is straightened by the arrival of a photon, your visual pigment is bleached. It loses its purple color and is unable to absorb light until it is reunited with another molecule of vitamin A with a bend at the elbow of its carbon chain. As you enter a darkened theater, ordinary sunlight may have completely bleached the pigment in your rods. Your fatter cones retain enough unbleached pigment to allow you to see the bright image projected on the screen, but they are not sensitive enough to react to the dimly lit row of seats next to you. Over the next several minutes, your rods will reassemble molecules of pigment with their bent carbon chains ready to spring straight once again, to translate the energy of the theater's dim light into the language of your brain and allow you to find an empty seat.

A carbon-chain spring amplifies the energy of the photon 1 million times. Nature is more than just efficient, she is downright frugal. You will be able to see a flash of light if only six closely spaced receptor cells each absorb a single photon. You will then need to reassemble only 6 of the 25 quadrillion molecules of visual pigment stored in the outer segments of your photoreceptor cells.

However, light perception is not vision. You may find it unsettling to learn that, to your eyes, the world is a senseless, two-dimensional montage of disconnected dots of light. Each dot appears to be equally far from you, equally important, and none even seems related to any other. This is a bit like what you would see if you were to place your nose against the canvas of a painting by the pointillist Georges Seurat. However, unlike those dried dabs of oil paint, the color of each point of light reaching your retina changes from moment to moment. To your photoreceptors, light reflected from the leaf of a tree might appear green, yellow, or red depending not on the season but on the intensity of the light reflecting from it, an intensity that can change from one minute to the next, an inconsistency your brain must resolve.

To add to the confusion, the image on the retina is inverted. Scientists in the sixteenth century were shocked when they made this disturbing discovery, and they struggled with the troubling implication that we see the world upside down. This so concerned Leonardo da Vinci that he postulated the existence of an additional lens in the eye that would revert the image to its upright position, one of his rare inaccuracies concerning human anatomy. This inverted image should have been a clue that you do not see with your eyes, but with your brain. This is more than just semantics. It is not that you somehow ignore this upside-down image or somehow adjust your orientation around it. You truly do not see it. You will see nothing until about one-twentieth of a second later. Even then, you will not see every point of light striking the retina, but only those that your brain found interesting and important. Photoreceptors collect confusion and, fortunately, you are completely unaware of that meaningless muddle of information stimulating your retina. Your brain, not your eyes, constructs your view of the world and it does this, literally, in the blink of an eye.

The neurophilosopher Daniel C. Dennett correctly observed, "Vision cannot be explained as a bottom-up, data-driven process; it requires expectations!"[2] Vision requires the memories and predictions that only your brain can provide. Your brain receives only sketchy reports that the retina has constructed from a confusing, constantly changing clutter of stimuli. It then fills in these minimalist sketches with the five ingredients necessary for vision: form, color, depth, motion, and meaning. Your brain makes ample use of memories to paint a vibrant, *useful* portrait of your surroundings.

There is one more incredible thing to consider. As they travel, photons have a mysteriously unified view of things. If they had taken a clock and an odometer with them on their trip from a distant star, the time and the distance traveled would have measured zero. At light speed, time stands still, distances collapse, and everything is here and now.[3] From the perspective of the photon, everything along its path—the star from which it came and you—exist at one point, simultaneously, and since time stands still, eternally. As you travel at your leisurely pace you are oblivious of that extraordinary state of affairs. Eternity and total unity are physical entities that lie outside of your direct awareness.

You are mindful only that those time-traveling bits of energy weave a rich, visual tapestry of your surroundings. Although it seems to be "out there" and separate from you, this colorful creation is embroidered entirely within your brain and is seamlessly interwoven with perceptions stitched by other senses. Even through closed eyes, it cloaks your memories, thoughts, and dreams.

5

The Intelligence
of the Neuron

Your Life Depends on the Decisions of Individual Cells

YOU WOULD NEVER KNOW about the signal of a photoreceptor if it did not join the chorus of literally trillions of electric impulses coursing through the substance of your brain. However, the signals from each rod and cone must audition for the chance to arrive on the stage of your awareness. Only a select few will see their name in lights. To make it, they have to convince a nearby *ganglion cell* to relay their signals down the optic nerve. It is here in the retina that your brain begins to weave your very subjective, visual version of reality.

Ganglion cells occupy the inner layer of the three-layered network of neurons that lines the inside of the eye. They communicate with the *photoreceptors,* the rods and cones in the outer layer of the retina, through an intermediate layer of *bipolar cells.*

89

Every rod and cone has a song for the ganglion cells to hear and, since there are about 125 photoreceptors for each ganglion cell, the intermediate layer of bipolar cells act as agents and arrange group auditions. Signals from a small group of rods and cones are presented to a ganglion cell that decides their fate, determining whether they will be silenced or sent down your optic nerve to join the choir of signals in your brain. The ganglion cell makes this selection without consulting you. Its decision depends quite literally on how the new notes harmonize with those around them.

Your brain is a collection of neurons, each making critical choices. These are individual, cellular judgments that you will have to live with. Stephen Kuffler, a brilliant physiologist who was particularly skilled in preparing neurologic specimens for laboratory experiments, was determined to learn how those important decisions are made. The ganglion cell in the retina of a cat seemed to be large enough to accommodate the electrodes that were available in 1953, and Kuffler hoped that it might be possible to record the signals of that arrogant neuron that determines on its own what you will eventually see. From these cells he was about to learn how a neuron makes the individual decisions that govern your life. In a basement laboratory at Johns Hopkins Medical Center, Stephen Kuffler opened the door to a Carnegie Hall filled with a music so unexpected and so revealing that researchers have been returning ever since, with steadily improving recording devices.[1]

The name Stephen Kuffler ought to be more widely known. The quality of his work and the force of his effervescent personality have profoundly influenced the course of neuroscience. With his rare blend of acumen, razor-sharp wit, easy affability, and gentle encouragement, he drew a succession of brilliant researchers to the small laboratory in Baltimore where he worked.

It would have been hard to predict Kuffler's academic success. He did not attend school until he was ten years old. Although he often seemed more interested in tennis than in textbooks, he excelled at whatever truly interested him. He won the Austrian tennis championship before his anti-Nazi activities and the fact that his maternal grandmother was Jewish were issues of much concern. After graduating from medical school in Vienna in 1938, it became clear that these would become grave matters, and he quickly immigrated to Australia. There, a chance game of tennis with Dr. John Eccles, a professor of physiology at Sydney University, changed his life. Kuffler's friendship with Dr. Eccles and Dr. Bernard Katz, both of whom later became Nobel laureates, led him into the little-known field of neurophysiology and, far more than any other individual, Stephen Kuffler stripped that field of its obscurity. His brilliant research led to academic posts at the University of Chicago, Johns Hopkins Medical School, and Harvard University where, by the time he was fifty-four years old, he was asked to form a new department, the department of neurobiology. Before 1967, the biology of the neuron had been studied only in the separate departments of biology, physiology, pharmacology, and anatomy. Kuffler quickly assembled a stellar group of like-minded scientists, including David Hubel, Torsten Wiesel, and Ed Kravitz, whose contributions to this story you will soon appreciate. Not much later, it could be said that the top academic positions in neuroscience throughout the world were held by Stephen Kuffler's former students. But at the age of forty, in a basement in Baltimore, he was focusing his attention—and a beam of light—on the retina of a cat.

When he had wired the ganglion cell for its first recording session, Kuffler expected that it would simply wait in hushed silence until the retina was stimulated with light. He was surprised to find that, without any light stimulus at all, the

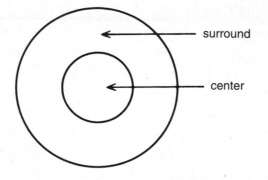

Figure 5.1   The ganglion cell's receptive field

ganglion cell produces a slow, irregular, continuous firing of impulses. Even more surprising, and terribly disappointing, there was practically no change in this spontaneous firing when he exposed the retina to light.

After checking and rechecking his instruments, Kuffler discovered that a ganglion cell will not respond to a spot of light unless it is so small that it illuminates only those photoreceptor cells within a small *receptive field* around it, an area usually less than one millimeter across. But Kuffler was further frustrated to find that the same stimulus got a different response from one trial to the next. A spot of light might elicit an "on response"—a burst of signals that sounds like vigorous applause for a bright spot of light, or slow, polite clapping for a dim one. On the next trial, the very same stimulus could produce an "off response"—a sudden decrease in the rate of firing or total silence, followed by a brief burst of signals as the light was turned off, as if to say, "Thank you, but that wasn't quite what we wanted." If this was an audition, it was not yet clear what the ganglion cell was looking for.

Kuffler's next finding held the answer. The ganglion cell's

receptive field, the small portion of the visual field that it pays attention to, is not treated as a simple circle. The ganglion cell divides its receptive field into two concentric parts, like a flattened doughnut. When the receptive field is lit, the ganglion cell's response to light coming from the "hole" is exactly opposite to its response to light coming from the surrounding doughnut it has baked from scratch.

Ganglion cells are looking for contrast. The ganglion cell compares the signals coming from the center of its receptive field with those coming from the area in the surrounding ring. If both parts are equally stimulated, as they were when Kuffler illuminated the entire retina with diffuse light, the ganglion cell will continue its slow, spontaneous firing as though nothing had happened. To excite the ganglion cell, there must be a significant contrast in the amount of light falling on those two areas of its receptive field. Only edges—the intersections of light and shadow—will do the trick.

When you look at a blank sheet of paper on your desk, millions of photoreceptors each report the intensity of the light of certain wavelengths coming from a single point of that image. Your ganglion cells ignore almost all of those reports. They pay attention only to those whose signals are different than those of their immediate neighbors, for example, where there is a contrast between light paper and dark wood. They alert you to the presence of the paper's boundary but tell you absolutely nothing about the contrast-free zone inside and outside of that border. The brain "fills in" the rest, painting uniform surfaces with the same color and brightness as the ganglion cells signal from their edges. The brain supplies form, color, depth, motion (or, in this case, the lack of it), and most important of all, meaning. It provides the "expectations" to which Dennett alluded. Your *eyes* report only about meaningless edges in a sea of confusion. Your *brain* sees a uniformly white, pliable, virginal piece of writing paper on a solid, wooden desk and con-templates the possibilities.

Your visual world is a mixture of light and dark surfaces, and scattered fairly evenly through the retina are two, cor-responding types of ganglion cells. In a remarkably efficient division of labor, an "on-center" ganglion cell responds most vigorously when more light falls on the center of its receptive field than on the surrounding ring, for example, bright spots against a dark background. "Off-center" ganglion cells respond most vigorously to dark spots on a bright background. If all ganglion cells were of the on-center type, small stars would make a greater impression on you than the letters on this page. Conversely, if you had only off-center ganglion cells, the night sky would lose its majesty.

Your perception of the size and shape of the letters on this page depends on the number and location of the off-center gan-glion cells in your retina that were persuaded to respond. The boldness of the letters depends on the frequency of their sig-nals. The greater the contrast, the faster they will fire. A dark letter printed on a white page will produce a more rapid burst of signals than will the same letter printed on gray or brown stationery. Fortunately, it is contrast rather than intensity that determines the frequency of a ganglion cell's firing; oth-erwise, you would be unable to read a book at the beach. Out-side on a sunny day, these letters would reflect so much light that, if the ganglion cells responded to intensity rather than contrast, the words would blend with this page and disappear. The organization of the ganglion cell's receptive field into antagonistic portions enables you to read as long as there is more than a 2 percent difference in the brightness of the page and its letters. It allows you to read indoors or out, by sun-light or by candlelight, and no, despite what you have been told, reading by candlelight will not hurt your eyes.

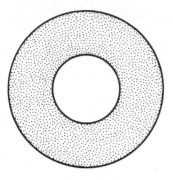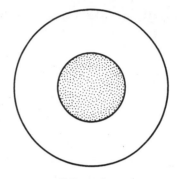

On-center
On-center ganglion cells respond to illumination of the center of the receptive field.

Off-center
Off-center ganglion cells respond to illumination of the surround.

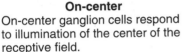

Figure 5.2   Two kinds of receptive fields

Even your ability to discriminate colors stems from the organization of the receptive field. Some ganglion cells fire only in response to contrasting borders of red and green and others only to borders of blue and yellow. With signals from the three flavors of cones, red, green, and blue, and these two types of ganglion cells, the brain is able to construct every color in the rainbow.

In the microscopic distance between the photoreceptors and the ganglion cells, the mind is already at work, making critical choices, finding sense in nonsense, creating order out of chaos. It ignores most of what you see and reports only about significant degrees of contrast and the wavelengths of preselected colors. The report that the ganglion cell sends down the optic nerve bears its own definition of reality with a strong bias built by evolution, a predilection for lines, bars, and edges.

Until 1953, our understanding of the brain was surprisingly consistent with that proposed by Immanuel Kant in 1781. In his *Critique of Pure Reason,* Kant divides mental faculties into the separate categories of sensibility—the passive collection of raw, sensory data—and understanding—the active, mental process that imparts meaning. Kuffler's cat gave us a vivid demonstration that sensibility and understanding are not as distinct as Kant and we had supposed. The ganglion cell begins the process of making sense of your surroundings. Although its simple reports about lines and edges will not take on their full meaning until they travel further through the brain, your understanding of the environment takes an important first step at this remote, sensory outpost. The two processes, sensibility and understanding, occur together in small, incremental steps. Their threads are thoroughly intertwined from the very beginning of their journey toward your conscious awareness, and they *both* gain sophistication along the way. Visual form is sculpted in one area of the brain; color, motion, and depth are added at others; and finally, contributions from still other areas provide the key ingredients of memory, meaning, and the added spice of emotion to complete a picture that can fully qualify as *vision*.

The enormous significance of Kuffler's work was not fully appreciated for another decade. He had demonstrated that the genius of the neuron lies in its ability to restrict its attention to particular signals and to ignore the rest. Every neuron throughout the brain has a *receptive field,* a specific group of neurons from which it receives its information, and each neuron has evolved its own rules as to the very specific input that will cause it to respond. A neuron in your spinal cord waits for a tap on your knee and signals your leg to kick, but it ignores a bruise of your shin or the smell of a rose. It will leave to other neurons the job of responding to those stimuli. There is a physical pathway connecting each neuron in your body to every other; however, signals do not pass helter-skelter through that complex maze. They move along pathways clearly defined by the anatomy of each neuron's branches and the chemical nature of each synapse. Each neuron has a sphere of influence. Each maintains a special relationship with certain cells with which it has established most-favored-neuron status. Understanding that the receptive field governs the behavior of the neuron was similar to learning that wind is caused by changes in barometric pressure and not by the whims of capricious gods. The brain was no longer an imponderable "black box."

The anatomy and chemistry of the receptive field dictate which of a neuron's neighbors will excite it, which will inhibit it, and to which it will be mildly indifferent. Patients with autism have difficulty understanding and communicating and they describe suffering from an excruciating barrage of exaggerated and disconnected stimuli. These symptoms reflect what can happen when the neuron loses its focus and escapes the single-minded constraint of its receptive field, when it no longer maintains its indifference to extraneous stimuli and it responds directly to signals that would normally lie well outside of its immediate awareness. The hallucinations of schizophrenia are the result of defects in chemistry, anatomy, or perhaps both, that intermittently disrupt receptive fields, allowing input from inappropriate sources in the visual and auditory cortex to take center stage. But this is getting ahead of our story and will be taken up in more detail in Chapter 10.

The retina is the brain's Rosetta Stone. It is where George Wald learned how neurons communicate with photons and begin our "quiet conversation with Nature," and it is where Stephen Kuffler discovered how other neurons begins to code that communication. It was also in the retina that John Dowling accepted the next major challenge. Dr. Dowling has devoted three decades of his brilliant career to learning how the signal of a neuron navigates through a neural network—how a messy tangle of neurons eventually conveys a coherent message.

John Dowling was a bright student at Harvard University studying the biochemistry of vision with George Wald, when he first read Kuffler's description of the ganglion cell's receptive field. He was already thinking of the retina as an *Approachable Part of the Brain,*[2] the subtitle of a textbook on the retina he was to publish years later. Dowling saw that, hidden within the complexity of the retina, was a golden opportunity to learn how the brain's networks of neurons are organized.

Kuffler's cat had posed a series of tantalizing questions: How do well defined, receptive fields arise out of the jumble of rods and cones in the retina? How does the retinal switchboard connect messages from 125 million photoreceptors to the one million ganglion cells that take only important calls? Later, computer models would provide some answers, but not even today's powerful computers can provide the solutions that Dowling and a few other intrepid souls discovered by diving directly into the seemingly hopeless tangle of the retina's layers of neurons. In 1964, John Dowling went to Baltimore as a junior member of the research team at Kuffler's old lab at Johns Hopkins Medical Center and started to unravel that Gordian knot.

In Tokyo that same year, Tsuneo Tomita at Keio University made a discovery so surprising that most of his contemporaries seriously doubted it. As strange as it seems, your photoreceptors are active only in the dark. Light turns them off! Until a photon arrives, large numbers of the photoreceptor's gated channels stay open and sodium ions enter the cell in sufficient numbers to cause it to send a slow, irregular stream of signals across its synapses. Light somehow shuts those gated channels and silences the cell. Dowling recognized this as a promising piece of his puzzle. It explained the surprising finding that the ganglion cells of Kuffler's cat were firing spontaneously in the dark even before he stimulated them. Paradoxically, it is the silencing of the photoreceptor, triggered by the arrival of a photon, which we perceive as light.

It would be some years before the cascade of molecular

events that explains this paradox would be discovered. In the process, we would learn how molecules store memories, form emotions, and direct the wiring of the brain. (You will have to wait only until the next chapter.) In the meantime, Dowling realized that, regardless of how the signal is generated, its path through the retina's tangled network respects a very precise blueprint. Like tracing the wires stuffed behind the wall plate of a telephone jack, understanding the neural connections in the retina would provide clues to the wiring of the rest of the brain, and having the wiring diagram of the brain would be crucial to learning how it works. Solving this puzzle would require combining the still separate study of the biochemistry of the neuron with the study of its physiology and anatomy.

After seven years in Baltimore studying the anatomy and electrophysiology of the retinal network, Dowling returned to Harvard in 1971 and brought a new emphasis on chemistry to the department of neurobiology. This fusion of neurophysiology, neuroanatomy, and neurochemistry was soon emulated at universities throughout the world and prompted those departments to join under a new name, neuroscience.

Prior to Dowling's work, the physiology of a neural network appeared to defy logic. Somehow, despite the *astronomical* numbers of their branching connections, the on-center pathways from photoreceptors, through bipolar cells, to on-center ganglion cells, remain separate and insulated from the off-center pathways. As if by magic, the right signal somehow gets to the right ganglion cell through a tangled web of neurons. By carefully correlating the chemistry of the synapses with their anatomical distribution, Dowling demonstrated how this magic is performed.

A huge leap in understanding the brain was made when it was discovered that each synapse is permanently endowed with transmitter chemicals and receptors that are either inhibitory or excitatory. The most common transmitter chemicals are *glycine* and *GABA* (gamma-aminobutyic acid), which inhibit a neuron by closing sodium ion channels and increasing its membrane potential; and *glutamate,* which excites the neuron by opening sodium ion channels and lowering its membrane potential toward the threshold for firing. By learning the specific chemical transmitters at each synapse along the way, Dowling could identify which ones would block the signal and which synapses would pass it along. By identifying the chemical character and distribution of these synapses, by finding which had glycine or GABA, and which had glutamate, one could follow the path of the signals through the retinal switchboard. This discovery was like finding that the telephone wires in your walls are color-coded. It meant that, with patience, the brain's communication network might be figured out.

Synapses create networks, and networks create patterns of signals that carry rich, meaningful messages. The result is a tapestry that is nothing less than your internal representation of the world around you; your ideas, your memories, your perceptions, and your behavior. Dowling showed us how these patterns are embroidered.

Sorting out the tangled web of neurons in the retina became a model for continuing brain research. John Dowling demonstrated the rich reward to be gained from bringing together separate disciplines of science. Soon a growing assortment of previous strangers would become collegial co-workers in university departments of neuroscience around the world. Computer scientists, biologists, chemists, and psychologists collaborated on brain research and soon began to realize that, like it or not, they were blurring the borders between science and philosophy. Their ranks were soon joined by full-time neurophilosophers such as Paul and Patricia Churchland, scholars with solid credentials in both of these spheres.

6

The Moving Parts of Your Brain

The Photon Illuminates the Lilliputian Machinery of the Neuron

ACTION REQUIRES MOTION. The interesting activities of everything from aardvarks to zebras and behaviors as varied as those of atoms, automobiles, and astronauts all depend on moving parts. For as long as the brain appeared to be motionless, the operation of that sedentary blob of tissue remained totally incomprehensible. The brain's mystery began to rapidly unravel only when we finally found its surprisingly dynamic machinery. The dynamo responsible for your activity is the well-rehearsed, gymnastic movement of agile molecules hidden within the neuron—and your operating instructions are written in those molecules as well. Trying to see these pulsing, thrusting, organic engine parts would be like standing in your backyard and looking for someone vigorously waving at you from the moon. They elude even the electron microscope. We have learned their shapes and studied their motion by showering them with X rays rather than with electrons or light. Within the brief span of a lifetime we have bridged the comparable distances to the moon and to the molecule, and we have touched them both.

With each passing day, we are growing increasingly familiar with the machinery in the neuron, an assembly of oddly shaped molecules of protein with family names such as *chemical messenger, G protein,* and *receptor enzyme,* and individual names too long to memorize. These molecules do not just sit there, nor do they simply float aimlessly in your protoplasmic, intracellular soup. They move purposefully. They wiggle, stretch, and twist by design. They perform their functions by *changing their shape* in very specific ways and in response to very particular cues, and their agility accounts for your own.

George Wald won the 1967 Nobel Prize by answering a metaphysical question with pure science. With great precision, he showed that you see not because of a powerful spirit emanating from your eyes, but because of the incredible delicacy of a molecule that quakes at the impact of a photon—predictably and reproducibly. Although he spoke poetically of discovering your "quiet conversation with Nature," what he had described was only the first word in that conversation. At that time, few seriously expected that we would ever go beyond that and learn the entire chain of events that begins with the realignment of a string of carbon atoms and ends with vision. But a small group of molecular biologists took up the challenge. Now calling themselves *molecular neurobiologists,* they entered the tiny world of the neuron to study the Lilliputian assembly of molecular machinery that performs the real work of the brain.

Like your own, the intelligence of the neuron derives from both external and internal sources. A nerve cell gathers information from its receptive field as well as from an inherited, internal owner's manual written in your DNA. Along that

102

twisted, double chain of nucleotides, coded in a four-letter alphabet (*g, a, t,* and *c,* for the organic bases guanine, adenine, thymine, and cytocine), is an absolutely original set of instructions for the design and production of your proteins—yours and yours alone. By breaking apart these proteins with enzymes, painstakingly analyzing the fragments, and reassembling them with recombinant DNA, researchers have pieced together one of nature's most complex puzzles. They have discovered the molecular bag of tricks that swings a neuron, and then you, into action.

The Tinkertoy-like diagrams of molecules in standard chemistry textbooks are misleading. H-O-H symbolizes a molecule of water; however, as you have seen with vitamin A, the shape of a molecule can make a big difference. The hydrogen atoms in a water molecule are held at a precise angle from the oxygen atom, producing a very specific, three-dimensional contour. The irregular, lumpy shape of water molecules accounts for their aggregation into icebergs that float rather than sink, and for water vapor that dissipates when heated. If the shape of the water molecule were only slightly different, this would be a barren planet with most of its water permanently frozen at the bottom of its seas, and enveloped by a thin, inhospitable atmosphere. A slight change in the shape of a molecule can mean the difference between life and death.

Protein molecules are made of amino acids strung together like beads in a necklace. The thousands of different proteins in your body differ from one another only in the kind, the number, and the order of the amino-acid beads in their chain. Only twenty kinds of amino acids are required to assemble every one of your proteins; however, they do not form conga lines spontaneously. Although they float about in abundance, amino acids latch on to each other only with explicit orders from your genes and in adherence to very strict rules. The visual pigment molecule has 348 amino acids arranged in a specific, coiled configuration. We know which amino acids they are, in what order they appear and, most important, the exact shape their string assumes once it is assembled and suspended in your photoreceptor cell. Of the three billion bits of instruction in your DNA molecule, all of the directions for assembling visual pigment are encoded on a single gene with 1,044 pairs of nucleotides, three for each of the 348 amino acids in the visual pigment molecule. This gene passed the precious gift of sight down from your distant ancestors and will present it to your grateful descendants.

You cannot survive for long without consuming some carbohydrate, fat, and protein (or the amino acids necessary to make protein). A kernel of rice contains almost all of the twenty amino acids your body needs to manufacture its proteins, and the remaining few are present in soy as well as in several other varieties of bean. It is no accident that rice and beans are the diet staple for much of the world's population. But even more urgent is your need for water. It is only when the molecules in your body are suspended in solution that they assume the varied shapes that give them purpose. To bring your molecules to life you must add water, a dash of salt, a pinch of vitamins and a sprinkling of minerals such as iron, calcium, zinc, and magnesium. When this mixture simmers at 98 degrees Fahrenheit, remarkable things happen.

In warm water, some parts of protein molecules clump together like fat droplets in a bowl of chicken soup. Other portions stick out like the spines of a caterpillar and would dissolve like sugar if not held to the rest of the molecule. Each amino acid in a long protein responds differently to water, either recoiling to avoid it or stretching out for a refreshing swim. It is the arrangement of these *hydrophobic* and *hydrophilic* amino acid components that sculpts the varied contours of your protein molecules. They determine, for example, that the tubular shape of an ion channel through the cell wall has exactly the right dimensions to accommodate a particular ion.

The shape of a protein molecule changes with variations in the attraction between key amino acids in its chain in response to electric or chemical cues. Protein molecules flip, flop, twist, or fold when the forces between their components change, just as your arm bends when you flex the muscles around your elbow. These gyrations cause ion channels to open and close and produce the signals of the neuron. They cause the vesicles in an

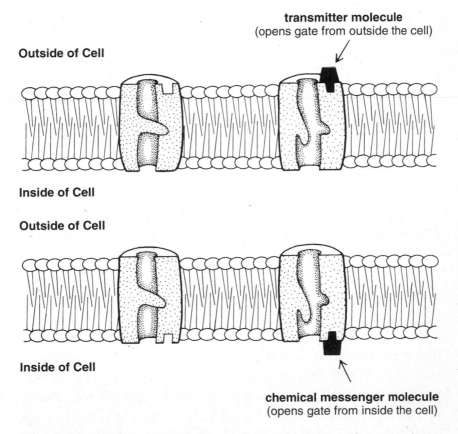

Figure 6.1 (Schematic) Two chemically gated ion channels: transmitter-gated and messenger-gated

axon terminal to burst at the synaptic membrane and discharge their chemical messengers, on cue, toward another neuron. Some particularly acrobatic molecules stretch, rotate and, like inchworms, carry developing axons and dendrites to new locations. Responding to specific electrochemical signals in their environment, they guide a growing nerve fiber like a slow-moving cruise missile, to the precise target in the brain where one particular neuron waits to make a critical synaptic connection with it. Molecules direct the wiring of the brain and produce the signals that travel those pathways. Undulating protein molecules are the fundamental elements of perception, and their tiny movements orchestrate all of your behavior. With this new perspective, the proteins that dot the neuron's membrane merit a closer look, a look that was not possible in George Wald's time.

Perhaps the simplest of these surface proteins, although simple hardly describes it, is the *voltage-gated ion channel*. It responds to a voltage reduction in the membrane around it by opening the passage through its tubular body just widely enough to allow an ion to pass through. Close relatives, *chemically gated ion channels,* are not moved by electrical events but, instead, open only with a proper, chemical key. Their amino acid chain is folded in such a way that one important crevice serves as a receptor site for a compatibly shaped neurotransmitter. Ion channels move quickly. It takes them one-thousandth of a second to open and they stay open for less than one-tenth of a second.

But you need to temper your responses to take into account your circumstances and base your immediate action on what has gone before. For this, your neurons are equipped with slower, more deliberate *nonchannel-linked receptors*. These proteins have no tubular opening into the cell. They are found only at the synapse, embedded in the wall of the receiving neuron with a receptor site on the outside of the cell and a tail projecting into the cell's interior (see Figure 6.2). When stimulated by

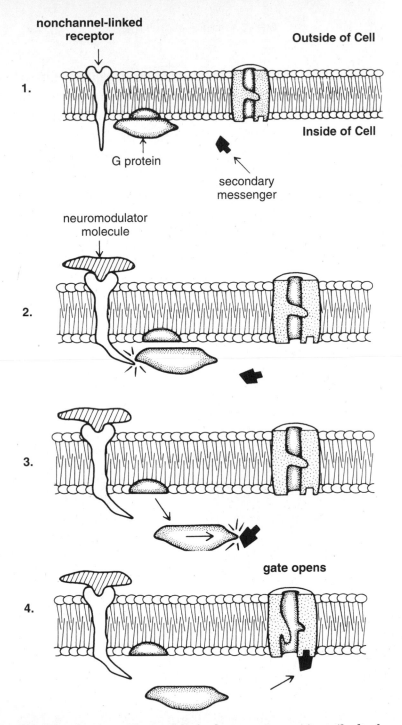

Figure 6.2 A nonchannel-linked receptor wags its tail, slowly

107

a transmitter chemical on the outside of the cell, this nonchannel linked receptor wags its tail to prod another protein on the inside of the cell, a G protein, into action. The G protein (the *g* stands for guanine, a chemical common to all members of this family) then moves about the cell to carry out the specific function it was instructed by your genes to perform. If all of this were blown up to toy-box proportions, Fisher-Price would have a wonderful new line and Disney could start a whole new series. The sluggish, tail-wagging nonchannel-linked receptor probably would not be as popular as its friskier, ion-channel neighbors. It may take as long as several seconds to react, and its

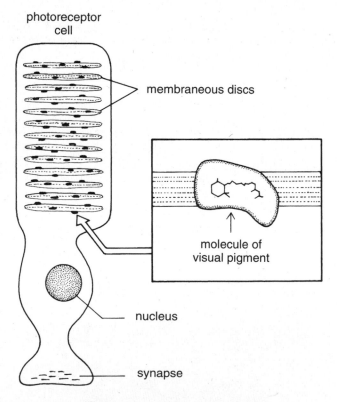

Figure 6.3 Visual pigment

tail sometimes takes minutes, hours, days, or even longer to return to its resting position. During that interval, the excitability of the neuron is altered, becoming either more reactive than normal or less so, depending on the particular molecules involved. Because of its ability to modulate the activity of the neuron, the chemical that activates a nonchannel-linked receptor is sometimes called a *neuromodulator* rather than a neurotransmitter. Neuromodulators first came to our attention because of the role that they play in Parkinson's disease and schizophrenia, and we have engaged them in chemical warfare using drugs such as L-dopa, thorazine, and Prozac. That war, and new drugs now under development, will be reported in Chapter 12.

George Wald had discovered only the beginning of a fascinating story. The arrival of a photon triggers a cascade of molecular activity that gains momentum like a tiny avalanche and yet proceeds with the precision of a well-planned military operation. In 1987, building on twenty years of prior work, a truly global group of researchers collaborating from laboratories in Moscow, Tokyo, Palo Alto, and Galveston deciphered the rest of that remarkable first sentence in our conversation with Nature. They described the well-oiled machine that a photon sets into motion.

The infinitesimal energy of a photon changes the shape of a *single* molecule of pigment, which causes the release of *dozens* of molecules of an enzyme, which cause the rapid breakdown of *hundreds* of molecules of a chemical messenger, which cause the gates in *thousands* of ion channels in the cell membrane to slam shut, which blocks *millions* of sodium ions from entering the cell, which produces the grand finale, a local change in the resting membrane potential. This electric event is your announcement that a photon has arrived. The exact nature of these enzymes, chemical messengers, ion channels and voltage

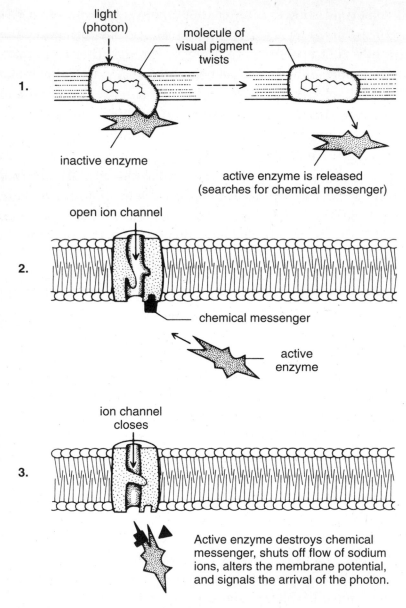

1. light (photon)

molecule of visual pigment twists

inactive enzyme

active enzyme is released (searches for chemical messenger)

2. open ion channel

chemical messenger

active enzyme

3. ion channel closes

Active enzyme destroys chemical messenger, shuts off flow of sodium ions, alters the membrane potential, and signals the arrival of the photon.

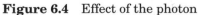

Figure 6.4 Effect of the photon

changes, and the precise roles they play in this brief performance, have been clearly identified.[1] But central to the whole event is the fact that *a molecule changed its shape.*

The 348 amino acids in a molecule of visual pigment are coiled into a roughly cylindrical blob. Embedded in this slightly lopsided structure is the bent carbon chain of vitamin A, made famous by Dr. Wald, waiting to be struck and straightened by a photon.

When the photon arrives, the straightening of that carbon chain produces a slight twist of the visual-pigment molecule. This subtle change is just enough to knock loose an enzyme that breaks up a chemical messenger, which shuts the sodium gates in the cell wall and creates the electric signal you see as light. This slight gyration also deprives the visual-pigment molecule of its purple color. It loses its light-absorbing property until its shape is restored by another bent carbon chain. With the arrival of another photon, this molecular ballet will be repeated.

It soon became apparent that the countless functions of the brain, even the formation of memories, are produced by variations of this intracellular, molecular choreography. In the late 1960s, a patient developed a peculiar form of amnesia after an injury to the hippocampus, a subcortical area of the brain bearing the Greek name for its sea-horse shape. Although she retained memories of events prior to her injury, she was unable to form new ones. To this intelligent and otherwise normal patient, the doctor who examined her on Monday was a total stranger on Tuesday. Each visit began with a poignant, one-sided charade of introductions. Several such patients demonstrated that one specific area of the hippocampus is necessary for the conversion of a current event into a memory you can store for a lifetime. We now have an idea as to how your hippocampus accomplishes this feat, and why hers did not.

When your doorbell rings and you ask "Who's there?," the muffled reply "It's me!" produces not only the auditory set of signals that you treat as symbols, but an emotional response as well. One set of signals identifies the speaker while another may fill you with delight, panic, or if you have never heard that voice before, bewilderment. Sensory signals that are linked with strong emotions or important associations get special treatment in the hippocampus and are stored for future recall. A special receptor found on neurons in one section of the hippocampus is ever on the lookout for this linkage of two sets of signals. This NMDA receptor is so named because it responds to N-methyl D-asparate as well as to glutamate. It is normally blocked by a magnesium ion and only in response to *simultaneous* stimulation from two separate sources will it release its magnesium lock and admit an extra influx of calcium ions into the cell. When the time interval between two signals is shorter than the lag between the signals of even the most rapid-fire neuron in the neighborhood, the NMDA receptor in the hippocampus lifts its magnesium blockade, allows extra calcium ions to enter the cell, and triggers a molecular ballet that tags this combination of signals with a claim ticket for future retrieval. It adds its own electric signature like a fingerprint, and marks this set of signals for future recall. It forms a memory.

In the course of a normal day's events, this receptor would ignore your chance sighting of an open door. However, in the daily routine of an escape-minded prisoner, the simultaneous perception of a door slightly ajar and the exciting thought of a flight to freedom will trigger a memory-inducing chain of molecular events. Today, an entire laboratory at Princeton University under the direction of Dr. Joe Z. Tsien is committed to studying this hippocampal receptor and the molecular events it sets into motion. They have come up with some startling findings.

When two signals simultaneously stimulate the NMDA receptors in the hippocampus and release its magnesium lock, the resulting influx of extra calcium molds a spaghetti-like molecule of protein, calmodulin, into the shape necessary to begin a reaction which, along with a number of related ones, are collectively referred to as *long-term potentiation* (LTP). This set of molecular events is now widely regarded as the neural basis for the formation of long-term memories.[2]

An increased concentration of calcium causes calmodulin to lose its random, wet-noodle configuration and stand up straight. It then joins a molecule with the catchy name calcium/calmodulin dependent protein kinase type II, which has been shyly waiting with its active site stuck to a portion of its own string of amino acids. Calmodulin presents the kinase molecule with a phosphate radical, a corsage containing one atom of phosphorus and four of oxygen. The kinase molecule extends her active site toward the calcium emboldened calmodulin, accepts the bouquet and together they begin to make memories. Their embrace produces a change in the electrical response of a hippocampal neuron. It causes the hippocampus to add a distinctive note marking a group of action potentials arriving at its dendrites as a distinctive, retrievable memory. These electrically tagged neurons will then maintain their ability to fire together as a group, and each time they do so, you will revive that stored memory.

The activated calmodulin molecule flips on the kinase switch of your memory. While kinase is in its extended configuration, the hippocampal neuron adds its own flourish to the current set of signals arriving from an associated group of neurons. When the kinase molecule loses its phosphate group, or is out of order because of injury or disease, your hippocampus will lose that ability. You will see everything as if for the first time and fail to learn the lessons necessary to survive.

In a recent, stunning experiment, Dr. Tsien at Princeton and several of his colleagues at MIT and Washington University isolated the specific gene that builds the hippocampal NMDA receptor, which initiates the memory-inducing chain of events called LTP. When given an extra copy of this gene, a group of mice grew extra NMDA receptors, and they learned and remembered better than their normal counterparts. They were able to find their way through a maze much more quickly and could perform a number of memory-related behaviors with far more proficiency than their normal litter mates.[3] Dr. Tsien was quoted in the *New York Times* confirming that it is now possible to genetically enhance intelligence and memory in laboratory mammals and he asserted that there is no reason to believe this could not be done in humans as well.[4] With gene therapy, we are on the threshold of helping patients suffering from memory loss and, before we have considered the ethical and practical consequences, we will be able to manipulate the intelligence of our offspring.

The molecular dances of calmodulin and kinase in your hippocampus, first noticed nearly three decades ago, are once again in the limelight and we now have the ability to exploit them. These molecules, which allow you to remember your phone number and to recognize a long-lost friend, perhaps will also help you to recall the main point of this chapter: The function of a molecule is determined by its shape. The changing contours of twisting molecules determine whether you will see, what you will remember, and how you will behave.

Actin is a molecule that behaves like an inchworm. Concentrated in especially large numbers at the end of a developing axon, it plays a major role in the wiring of the brain. As a young axon grows toward its destination, its trip is guided by a *growth cone,* an actin-rich swelling at its leading tip that behaves like the sophisticated guidance system in the nose of

114

a smart bomb. The growth cone is attracted to some chemical and electrical signals in its surroundings and is repelled by others. Using these clues, and propelled by molecules of actin, it unerringly leads the developing axon to a specific target. The growth cone guides an axon from your developing eye or toe to the precise neuron in your brain that waits to join with it and form an appropriate synapse.

Santiago Ramón y Cajal was intrigued by these swollen tips of immature axons on his microscope slides. Even though he could not see them move, he correctly imagined them behaving like "a battering ram, endowed with exquisite chemical sensitivity, rapid amoeboid movements, and certain impulsive force, thanks to which it is able to proceed [toward] its final destination." Cajal was a self-proclaimed romantic who would have preferred to follow his talents as an accomplished painter, but became a physician to please his father. The following passage is a wonderful insight into the mind of this nineteenth-century pioneer as he wondered about the life of the neuron. "What mysterious forces precede the appearance of these prolongations, promote their growth and ramification, and finally establish the protoplasmic kisses, the intercellular articulations that appear to constitute the final ecstasy of an epic love story?"[5]

One hundred years after Cajal first speculated about these intimate events in the life of a neuron, textbooks continue to adopt an incredulous tone when describing the growth cone. Otherwise dry textbooks lapse into colorful descriptions of the growth cone as it "continuously and exuberantly explores its environment, changing its shape, advancing first in one direction and then the other, sometimes splitting into diverging branches. Fingerlike projections from its sides and leading edge continuously expand and retract, and sheets of cell membrane alternately protrude or retreat backward over the surface of the growth cone as ruffles."[6] The uncanny activity of the growth cone depends on the interaction of two protein molecules, actin and myosin—the same two molecules that cause your muscle to contract. Aggregated in large numbers in your arms and legs, they can literally move mountains. In your developing brain they move the delicate branches of your nerve cells.

The molecules in your brain create its magic. They initiate the signals of the neuron and create the pathways they will follow. With equal ease, they can produce the twitch of an eyelid or the plans for a nuclear reactor. And yet, like voters, each molecule casts a single ballot not knowing what the cumulative outcome will be. The momentous consequences of its action lie far beyond its tiny realm.

Beta-secretase is a molecule whose actions have wrenching ramifications. It begins a process that, long before its fatal conclusion, slowly steals the memories of its victims and destroys their sense of who they are. Alzheimer's disease is far more common today (an estimated 12 million cases worldwide) than in 1907, when the German physician Alois Alzheimer first noted its distinctive, pathological signature. In the shrunken brain of a deceased patient, he found scattered, microscopic deposits of a substance called amyloid. A second feature, tangled fibers in many of the nerve cells, was noted later. These minute changes are devastating to the brain, to its hapless owner, and to the family that is left with an invalid stranger who looks exactly like their loved one but who neither recognizes them nor acknowledges their continuing care and concern. This process may begin with a single enzyme, beta-secretase. Enzymes are proteins that work in every tissue in your body. They usually either break apart other proteins or join them together. They are snippers or glue-ers. Beta-secretase is a snipper and it has a predilection for snipping at a harmless molecule of protein, an amyloid precursor, which hangs off the surface of many neurons like a string on a balloon. When beta-secretase snips off a section of this protein, the cast-off bit, a short chain of amino acids, joins with others just like it to form plaques of amyloid, which seem to gradually gum up the works. However, amyloid plaques do no harm to normal neurons and, even in Alzheimer's disease, only some neurons are affected. Another molecule, Apolipoprotein E3 (ApoE3), is thought to be protective.[7] The ApoE3 molecule is essential for the construction of micro-tubules that carry vital nutrients through the neuron. In the absence of ApoE3, these tubules seem to be susceptible to the toxic effects of amyloid; they lose their integrity and collapse, forming useless tangles. The absence of one specific molecule may lead eventually to the death of the neuron and to an inex-orable loss of memory, of personality, and of life itself. In the performance of your amazing orchestra of neurons, a broken string and a dissonant note cause more than just a bad review.

In 1997, the critical role of ApoE and its correlation with the risk of developing Alzheimer's disease was confirmed, and a test for the gene that makes that molecule was developed. However, since not everyone who tests positive gets the disease, a positive result could lead someone to misinterpret normal forgetfulness and to make inappropriate, life-altering decisions. Knowledge of an increased risk could also lead to premature or inappro-priate actions by employers and insurance companies. Until there is an effective treatment, this test is available only as additional confirmation of the diagnosis of Alzheimer's disease in people with unmistakable symptoms of dementia. If treat-ment and prevention become possible, this test or others like it will be used to identify those who would benefit.

The first step toward a cure and prevention is identifying the broken bits of machinery that lead to such tragic ends. In 1999, after a ten-year search, scientists at Amgen, a biotech-nology company in Thousand Oaks, California, identified and isolated the enzyme beta-secretase and the search is on for a drug to block it.[8] A test for genetic susceptibility to Alzheimer's disease and an effective means of preventing it could mean that our children might know of this dreaded disease only in the way that we remember smallpox and polio.

In the years since we discovered how a molecule converts the energy of the photon into the language of the neuron, the brain's machinery has became accessible. We have learned to navigate and work in a world measured in nanometers. The astonishing, practical implications of this new capability led molecular biologists to join with bioengineers, entrepreneurs, and venture capitalists. Research suddenly moved into a new environment. Companies in Silicon Valley acquired academicians from their ivory towers and dramatically changed our view of the future. These joint adventurers are mobilizing enormous financial, technical, and intellectual resources. Their mission statement is nothing less than to understand and master the forces that orchestrate the life-and-death dances of your molecules.

A new science, *proteomics,* has emerged. Entrants into this new field of protein research are automating the process of analyzing proteins in an effort to more rapidly identify the causes of disease and speed up the process of developing new therapies. Keith Yamamoto, chairman of cellular research at the University of California at San Francisco, has characterized this new science as a revolution similar in magnitude to *genomics,* the race to map the billions of bits of information coded in your DNA. Proteomics will make it possible to study all of the proteins designed by your DNA and to analyze the components, structure and shape of each of them, in health and in disease. In minutes, simply by placing minute tissue samples into a device no bigger than a bread box with scales able to weigh individual molecules and lasers capable of detecting their shape, technicians can produce images of molecules that are far more accurate than the rough approximations, which previously were the imperfect results of months of difficult, labor-intensive laboratory work.

As clearly as the steam engine and cotton gin marked the beginning of the industrial revolution, these enterprises are the harbingers of a biotechnical revolution that will dwarf its predecessors. Fulfilling the promises of this revolution will require a clear understanding of how the brain's signals are produced by individual molecules, how they travel through single neurons and spread across your vast, exquisitely coordinated networks of neurons—which leads us back to the yellow brick road.

7

The Yellow Brick Road

To Your Biological Clock and Internal Maps of the Universe

So FAR WE HAVE CONSIDERED how ions and molecules create signals that differentiate the neuron from every other living cell. It is the orchestration of those signals that distinguishes you from everyone else, even from your identical twin if you happen to have one. To find out how trillions of neural signals are organized into the patterns that create your individuality, it is necessary to trace their connections and follow their pathways. We need a road map.

In 1968, Tony Stretton and Ed Kravitz at Harvard University's newly formed Department of Neurobiology quite literally followed a yellow road into the intimidating network of the brain's neurons. They injected a fluorescent dye into the cell body of a single neuron and watched the greenish yellow chemical being transported along its axon and through all of its dendrites. For the first time it was possible to accurately trace the branches of a particular neuron through the forest of its neighbors. A more high-tech method was soon developed for marking a trail through that forest. *Autoradiography* cleverly causes selected cells to photograph themselves. By bathing neurons with radioactive amino acids and exposing them to a photographic film, those neurons that absorb the labeled molecules and pass them across synapses to their neighbors produce a beautiful photograph showing which neurons actively communicate with which others. As neurons pass these radioactive chemicals from one neuron to the next, they create a perfect self-portrait of a neural circuit.

Brand-new maps of the brain were drawn based on the chemistry and connections of its individual neurons, and the visual pathway took some surprising turns. Some of the ganglion cells in the retina were found to send their axons to an area of the brain that has nothing to do with vision. This area proved to be the long-sought timekeeper of the brain, your biological clock.

Nearly all living organisms keep time. The pervasive rhythms of activity in plants and animals are not just a passive response to cycles of night and day, they are innate. In the sixteenth century, Carolus Linnaeus, famous for his classification of plants and animals into phyla, orders, and species, created a "clock garden." He planted a variety of carefully selected flowers that open their petals on such precise, individual schedules that he could accurately tell the time just by looking at his blossoms. Two centuries later, in 1729, the French astronomer Jean Jacques d'Ortous de Mairan noted that his plants, which opened their leaves during the day and closed them at night, would open them again in the morning even when they were kept in total darkness. Bees arrive at a source of sugar water at the same time every day, and in the early 1900s, Karl von Frisch and Ingeborg Beling found that they keep precisely to their schedule even when their hives are placed deep in a salt mine isolated from any external time cues. In 1955, Gustav Kramer and Klaus Hoffman demonstrated that starlings orient themselves toward their destination and time their flight using internal cues, which persist in the dark and are only slightly modified by the local environment. Anyone who has traveled rapidly through several time zones can attest to the disruption caused by the difference between the local time and the time measured by their internal clock.

Your biological clock is a small cluster of neurons called the *supra-chiasmatic nucleus* (SCN), just above (supra) the crossing junction (chiasm) of the optic nerves, where one-half of the axons from each eye pass to the opposite side of the brain. It is nestled near the pineal gland and the pituitary gland, which synchronize their secretions with its ticking. The SCN periodically resets its timing mechanism using information from the retina about the length of the day. It gets this data from axons discovered with autoradiography, axons that leave the optic nerves at the chasm just below. These axons do not signal about contrast, as do those going to the visual cortex; they signal only about the ambient level of light. The SCN passes this information to the pineal gland, which modulates its secretion of melatonin, producing more of this hormone at night than during the day.

The pituitary gland is also lulled into following the rhythmic signals from the SCN and causes nearly all of your body's other hormones; your immune, cardiovascular, urinary, and reproductive systems; and nearly every aspect of your physiological and emotional life to get in step with this circadian rhythm (circa = approximate; dia = day). This rhythm can be monitored directly in the daily rise and fall of your body temperature and your renal activity, both of which are highest in the early evening and lowest right before awakening, and in your adrenal gland's output of cortisol and aldosterone, which peak in the early morning and are lowest at bedtime. Your body knows what time it is even when you don't.

The brain really does tick. Signals do not travel through it instantaneously, but rather at measured intervals. It takes a small but specific part of a second to appreciate pressure, pain, and sound because signals have to traverse sensory circuits, each of which has a specific transit time. For the visual pathway this is one-twentieth of a second. You are totally oblivious to those events occurring outside of the time frame that the wiring of your brain has set. Black bars pass across a movie screen between individual frames too quickly for you to notice. Glaciers grow far too slowly. If wired with far greater complexity and much longer conduction times, your brain might see the sun and stars as they might appear in time-lapse photography, racing across a sky blinking alternately black and blue, and you would never notice a passing butterfly.

The staccato, flitting movements of most birds indicate that their internal clocks tick much faster than yours. During the brief moment when you see a flash of color diving into a thorny thicket, they find the time to choose a safe landing site and alight delicately on a carefully selected twig. They see insects, cats, and people moving as if in slow motion, and they hear whole melodies in a single chirp. Like a metronome, the fixed conduction times of the circuits in the brain mark time. They regulate the rhythm of your movements, the lilt and timing of your speech and the tempo of the music that you will produce and enjoy. The ticking of your brain creates a river of related events and establishes its rate of flow. Tapping out the pace and rhythm of your life, it gives you your inescapable sense of passing through time.

Einstein proved that time and space are one, but your brain

treats them separately and gives each a new meaning. It divides where from when and separates beginning from middle and end. From your perspective, a meteorite momentarily streaks the summer sky. Rose petals open slowly, performing a protracted passion play with continually changing colors and fragrance, until they finally fall. Yet all the while, the invisible stuff of which meteors and flowers are made, their clouds of subatomic particles, remain oblivious and untouched by these seemingly spectacular events. If asked, they might say with incredulity, "Did we do that? We had no idea! Let us tell you what it looked like from here." Unchanged, they continue to spin through space/time, a physical dimension you cannot truly fathom.

Your human perspective gives new shape and meaning to particles beyond your ken. Like sculptures in the clouds, your brain forms memories of gossamer events, cloaks them with attributes of your own making and marks them with your personal sense of time. For as long as it keeps ticking, the timepiece in your brain senses a before and an after, and causes you to care deeply about the difference.

Your biological clock ticks away in the darkness of your skull and, but for its connection with your retina, would keep you to a daily cycle about twenty-five hours long. That is not a misprint. You were born with a twenty-five-hour, not a twenty-four-hour clock. People who are deprived of periodic daylight because of blindness or by being confined to an environment with an unchanging level of light, wake up about an hour later each day if they are not disturbed. The light of a new day resets your errant internal clock. It continuously adjusts your body's rhythms to the planet's rhythmic exposure to the sun—even as that period of sunlight varies with the season. When you globe hop, your brain lags behind. Gradually, as signals from your retina reset your internal clock to match the periods of daylight in your new time zone, your pituitary gland reins in your hormones, your metabolism gets back on schedule, and you begin to feel yourself again.

The technique of autoradiography, photographing axons as they transmit labeled chemicals along their neural circuits, confirmed that the vast majority of ganglion cells send their reports to the visual cortex, the area at the back surface of the brain that is directly concerned with vision. But this trip is not a direct one, and it ends with a surprise. Those photogenic, radioactive molecules pass down the ganglion-cell axons through the optic nerve to the chiasm and, after negotiating this crossing junction, end in the thalamus. This is a paired, egg-shaped group of nuclei, one half sitting on each side of the brain just below the cortex. The thalamus (Greek for chamber) is the brain's Ellis Island, a central clearing house where nearly all sensory signals are gathered as they arrive from every part of your body before being sent on to fulfill their potential in the cortex. In each half of the brain, axons from one half of each retina end in a part of the thalamus devoted exclusively to vision, the lateral geniculate nucleus (LGN). There, they pass their sensory signals like so many batons to be carried by the neurons of the LGN for the second leg of the trip, from the thalamus to the visual cortex. When these thalamic axons arrive at the cortex, autoradiography shows that they are organized in a manner that would challenge the finest marching band.

In your developing brain, 1 million embryonic axons arrive at each half of the visual cortex in a bundle, carrying a messy mixture of signals from both retinas. Immediately, these axons separate into alternating rows at the back of your brain, each band carrying signals exclusively from either the right eye or the left. For their astonishing grand finale, within these alternating rows, the axons arrange themselves so that each axon terminal in the visual cortex exactly replicates the relative position of the ganglion cell in the distant retina from which its report originated. The result is that adjacent points of light in your environment send their signals to adjacent points in your visual cortex. Like placard-carrying members of a marching band spelling out the name of their team, the axon terminals at the back of each half of your brain produce a map of the opposite half of your visual world.

To appreciate this engineering feat, David Hubel has suggested a mental exercise that I will paraphrase: For a moment, imagine that you enlarge the retina and the brain so that the ganglion cells become as large as peas. Then imagine that, from each eye, you gather about half a million of their axons into a cable reaching to the thalamus, a distance equal to the length of a football field. There, you splice each axon to another neuron whose axon reaches the length of a second football field, to the visual cortex. Now you are asked to arrange the far ends of those second axons in precisely the same relative position as the million, pea-sized ganglion cells now out of sight in the retina two hundred yards away. Neighboring axons must report from neighboring ganglion cells. And you are not finished yet. Both eyes have to be represented in this map. Binocular vision and depth perception require that next to each axon reporting from your right eye, you must place an axon that reports from exactly the same relative position in the left eye.

There is simply not enough room in the genetic code to direct such a complicated task. The trillions of connections in the brain far outnumber the three billion bits of instruction in your DNA. Heredity provides only a general plan, laying down rough pathways marked by glial cells. But we now have a clue as to how axons get the rest of their specific marching orders. They are given step-by-step instructions from their immediate neighbors. They give each other subtle clues that lead each one to its precise, final location, where it will find its compatible mate and form a proper synapse.

This surprising discovery was made in the retina of the developing fetus of a cat. As the embryonic ganglion cells begin their slow, irregular, seemingly random firing, Carla Shatz and her co-workers at Stanford University noticed that they fire synchronously with their immediate neighbors more often than they do with cells farther away. In this subtle way, embryonic ganglion cells develop an affinity for their earliest companions. As they mature and begin their journey through the brain, axons travel with the axons they "got to know" in their infancy.[1] An electrical and chemical conversation with their earliest neighbors guides them along their route. Those subtle, electrochemical signals lead them like so many guided missiles to their precise, distant destinations. The amazing precision of their connections insures that the back of your brain has an accurate map of your visual universe. For an animal that moves about, the accuracy of that map is essential for survival.

Other visual maps have been found crammed into small crevices and etched onto tiny bumps in the brain. Some ganglion cells send their axons to form miniature visual maps on two tiny lumps, the *superior colliculi,* on either side of the midbrain. Here, they connect with the neurons that move your eye muscles so that your eyes will make an instantaneous, automatic jump toward an unexpected change in your visual environment. When a door is silently but *suddenly* opened at the side of a conference room in the middle of an important meeting, many sets of eyes will move in that direction—in unison, instantly, and involuntarily. This reflex does not involve the visual cortex. It will occur even after a totally blinding injury to the back of the brain. Amazingly, patients with severe, bilateral damage to the visual cortex (a rare cause of blindness) still accurately move their eyes toward suddenly moving objects because of unseen signals from their retinas to their superior colliculi. These are the same nuclei responsible for the frog's uncanny ability to snag a fly on the wing. Even though a frog has fairly poor vision by our high standards, some of its ganglion cells respond to the distinctive size and shape of a flying insect the way ours do to lines and edges. The signals from those ganglion cells do not go to the frog's primitive visual cortex, but to its superior colliculi, which accurately direct its tongue to a vaguely seen target.

Those maps on the superior colliculi are interesting for another reason. They demonstrate the efficient engineering of the brain: No neuron is indispensable. Your brain never depends on any single neuron, but only on the accumulated effects of large numbers of them. The speed of the reflex movement produced by the superior colliculus is determined by the *average* speed of the firing of all of the neurons in that little bump. The new direction of your gaze (or of the frog's darting tongue) is dictated by the *location of the center of the active group* in that collection of neurons. Here as elsewhere in your brain, the loss of an individual neuron will have an imperceptible effect.

More than fifteen such topographical maps have since been discovered in the brain. They represent the tactile, auditory, olfactory, and every other sensory aspect of your world, both inside and outside of your body. Finding these maps and learning their function has been a bit like the experience of painting by numbers. After a few areas are filled in, a meaningful pattern begins to emerge. The maps that have emerged on the convoluted surface of the brain suggest that it is expressly organized to create its own facsimile of the universe, a facsimile whose appearance is determined by the nature of your sense organs, and whose limits are dictated only by what you can imagine.

8

The Emerald City

The Secrets of the Most Complex Functions of the Brain

THE VISUAL CORTEX at the back surface of the brain is often described as the jeweled screen upon which your visual world is somehow projected. When David Hubel and Torsten Wiesel joined Stephen Kuffler at Harvard University, they were the first to enter this dazzling theater. Both of them had worked with Kuffler in Baltimore and were delighted to join him when he was invited to be a professor of pharmacology at Harvard. Later, they were part of the enthusiastic young group of researchers that formed his new department of neurobiology. By then, the signals of the ganglion cell had been traced to the back of the brain and had been well-studied at points along that route. Hubel and Wiesel devised a way to record the signals of individual neurons in the visual cortex that receive those signals, and they changed the course of neuroscience. With tungsten electrodes—much finer than Kuffler had used in the retina—placed into a single, cortical neuron of a cat, they learned the fascinating process by which the brain organizes your sensations.

Cortical neurons are small. When viewed under a microscope, they compare to ganglion cells as grains of sand compare to kernels of corn. And yet, their diminutive size holds a much greater degree of complexity than Kuffler had found in the ganglion cell. Hubel and Wiesel's cat, after undergoing delicate microsurgery to implant a state-of-the-art electrode in its brain, walked about unbothered, purring, and behaving normally. Then, as it looked at tiny, illuminated targets, it made history. Recordings from its visual cortex revealed how cortical neurons begin to transform a bewildering barrage of sensations into useful, meaningful perceptions.

The Hubel and Wiesel experiments inspired new generations of researchers with a powerful demonstration that even the most complex functions of the brain could be made understandable. When they were awarded the Nobel Prize in 1981, one year after the death of their friend, colleague and mentor, Stephen Kuffler, no one could have imagined the degree to which their work would accelerate the pace of brain research. Their success inspired others to follow the signals from the cerebral cortex to neurons in nearly every part of the brain.

The picture that Hubel and Wiesel found projected on the visual cortex is a mosaic. Each small fragment is projected and processed independently. The intricate details of each piece are composed in isolation from the rest. There is no sense of wholeness here. The visual cortex is a kaleidoscope where small, independent groups of cortical neurons busily edit and richly embellish piecemeal reports from the ganglion cells, gracing each with form, depth, color, and motion. They do this all within a matter of milliseconds, yet well before you will understand this composition.

Hubel and Wiesel began their work with a comic parody of Kuffler's earlier experience. Even though they used a suitably small spot of light to stimulate the retina, they were unable to excite the neuron in the visual cortex from which they were recording. After repeated, unsuccessful attempts, a previously unnoticed crack in a projection slide ended their frustration and gave them their first lucky clue as to what goes on in this, as yet unexplored, area of the brain. Only when the cracked slide was moved across the beam of projected light did their electrode record a brief response. In this inelegant way, Hubel and Wiesel discovered that some of the cells of the visual cortex respond only to edges moving across their receptive field. Testing neighboring neurons led to the astonishing discovery that some neurons respond only to vertically oriented lines, others only to horizontal ones, and others only to edges oriented in a very specific direction in between. Some cortical neurons respond only to lines of a specific length or width, some only to edges that form corners or curves and some only to borders that move in a specific direction. The neurons in the visual cortex demonstrate a staggering degree of individual specialization, and they are distributed in a highly organized manner.

The cerebral cortex, the brain's thin, outer covering, is a quiltwork of patches. Each tiny patch is a column of six distinct, parallel layers of neurons. They are usually no more than one millimeter across and extend the full thickness of the cortex—pegs of brain cells no wider than a pinhead and only two or three millimeteres long. These patches are invisibly stitched with synapses and are distinguished only by their separate functions. Hubel and Wiesel confirmed that the visual cortex is a collection of approximately one thousand of these modular columns of cells. Within each tiny column is the machinery necessary to extract recognizable features from one small portion of your visual world.

Like prospectors panning for gold, each of the columns in the visual cortex filters a tiny portion of the stream of signals flowing through and collects small nuggets that may hold meaning. Each column passes along a set of electric spikes whose rhythm and syntax ascribe visual attributes to one fragment of your world.

The complexity of these six-layered module far exceeds that of the three-layered switchboard in the retina. Each column in the visual cortex receives approximately five thousand retinal reports about borders, edges, and contrast differences. Each column then sends out about fifty thousand reports of its own, encoded with richly embellished descriptions of the size, shape, orientation, and movement of those borders, their position in your visual field, the wavelengths of their light, and their position and distance relative to you and to each other. This is a far cry from the completely formed image some had expected to find projected on the visual cortex, but it is a most efficient way of creating one.

The action potentials leaving the occipital cortex are coded with all of the necessary elements to compose a useful picture, but you still do not "see" it, and if you did, it would make no sense. The visual cortex creates thousands of exquisitely formed pieces of a puzzle. The rest of the brain has to put them together.

Attempts have been made to enable the blind to see by sending electric signals to the visual cortex from a miniature camera mounted on a pair of glasses.[1] The video image was transformed into electric stimuli in a computer worn on the belt and sent through an array of microscopic electrodes permanently implanted in the brain.

Patients with permanently blinding eye disorders, who had this surgery several years ago, report that the vision they regained was very limited and a far cry from normal vision, producing diffuse flashes of light rather than meaningful images. However, after a period of intensive training, they were able to walk unaided, use public transportation, watch television, and use a computer.

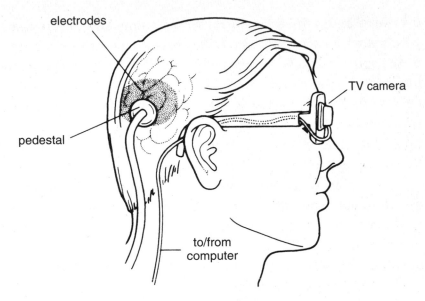

Figure 8.1 Artificial vision

For procedures like this to be more successful, it will be necessary to accurately plug very large numbers of electrodes, point for point, into precisely chosen layers and columns of cortical neurons. This amazing technology is in its infancy and its potential is staggering. At its heart is the insight that Hubel and Wiesel gave us into the remarkable organization of the cerebral cortex.

YOUR BRAIN CRAVES PATTERNS and searches for them endlessly. In the absence of adequate sensory input, it will even make its own. Under conditions of severe sensory deprivation, the brain will create homemade patterns, which may take on a bizarre, hallucinatory character. In some African villages, young men destined for the tribal priesthood are introduced to the spirit world with initiation rites that include being left buried up to their necks in sand with their eyes and ears covered until they experience such hallucinations. The apparitions produced under these stressful conditions are often quite terrifying and, out of each large group of initiates, only one or two persevere to become shamans.[2]

Under normal circumstances, the cerebral cortex receives a continuous wave of sensory signals. With its thousands of modular columns of cortical neurons, it breaks up that flow of visual, tactile, auditory, and olfactory information into manageable, bite-sized pieces and looks for clues to its meaning. While this process has obvious survival value, distinguishing predator from prey in the wild, or identifying hazards in your home and workplace, your cortex continues to sift through sensory morsels even in the secure surroundings of the concert hall and art gallery, purely for pleasure. Each tiny, cortical module savors and scrutinizes associated groups of signals as if collecting shards of broken pottery in an archaeological dig. Their fragmentary reports are compared, contrasted, and fit together in various ways that produce reactions throughout the brain. Signals that evoke an "Ooh!" or an "Ah!" will trigger molecular events in the hippocampus that produce memories. In other subcortical areas, they may set into motion molecular dances that produce revulsion, joy, or rapture. Digesting sensory stimuli is just as necessary and often just as satisfying as consuming a good meal.

A newborn infant seems not to see very much, and this was once believed to be a sign that its retina is not developed as fully at birth as we now know it to be. You initially seemed disinterested in your visual world simply because vision requires memories, and on the first day of your life that was something you sorely lacked. The shapes around you may have been mildly entertaining but, with one important exception, they were completely meaningless and evoked little response. That exception was the human face. A newborn will ignore excitedly waving hands and expectantly offered toys, but the full, frontal view of a nearby face invariably gets attention. The easiest way to assess the visual acuity of an infant is to position yourself at close range and see if it will turn to follow as you move your head slowly and deliberately across its field of view. Within minutes of delivery, having never seen a face before, a neonate will selectively turn toward even a crude, cardboard pattern that merely hints of two eyes, a nose, and a mouth—as long as those elements are in approximately the correct relation and proportion. Knowledge of the significance of that pattern appears to be inborn. Newborn chicks also have an inherited response to patterns never seen before. The Dutch ethologist Nickolaas Tinbergen found that chicks raised in isolation, having never seen a hawk, crouched, cried, and ran for cover when presented with a silhouette of the shadow of that natural predator. Similar shadows of geese, ducks and other innocuous birds of similar size produced no unusual behavior.[3] Adding to a sparse, inherited collection, the brain learns to recognize a growing number of significant patterns, to associate them with meaning, and to attach appropriate responses.

Sounds, too, are constantly filtered for patterns that might have meaning. A visiting Eskimo would at first hear spoken English as an infant does, as a continuous string of gibberish. Instinctively, you would communicate to your foreign guest as you would with a small child, by exaggerating the pauses between your words and the inflections and gestures that accompany them. Sifting through that punctuated noise, the untutored brain will eventually recognize some patterns of sound as useful symbols and begin to draw meaning from them.

135

Even random noise is always scanned for a familiar voice or a remembered melody. Several times each second, the six layers of cells spread so vulnerably over the surface of your brain sift through the sands of sensation in search of the building blocks of language, memories, music, any stray pieces that might be used to make sense of the world and minimize its risks. Vibrations from the ground, flashing lights, and the whistle of a train enable you to evaluate your present situation, predict the future, develop a plan, and execute behavior that will let you survive a little longer in your rapidly changing environment. Starting with the uncoordinated attempt of an infant to reach, touch, and taste, the brain continuously updates its impressions of the world outside of you, the world within, and the interface between the two. From these, it builds a collection of electric patterns, reproducible neural tapestries leading to symbol recognition and complex thought.

The exploration of the visual cortex did more than give us our first glimpse of the complex mechanisms underlying perception. Hubel and Wiesel blazed a trail that would disclose how memories are triggered, stored, and retrieved, how threats and opportunities are evaluated, and how we plan and execute our behavioral responses. They also produced the first hard evidence that your experiences shape the brain, adding scientific fuel to the ongoing debate about the relative importance of nature and nurture.

The roles played by heredity and the environment in making a human being have been hotly debated for centuries. In the 1600s, John Locke revolutionized educational and political thought with his description of the child's mind as a blank slate, placing unprecedented responsibility upon those in charge of their upbringing. That liberal view was hotly contested and, by the end of the nineteenth century, with growing awareness of

Mendel's laws of heredity, the pendulum had swung to the opposite pole.

Sigmund Freud's radical contention that behavior is shaped by experience ran completely counter to the widely held conviction of his day. Freud grew up in a world whose most respected scholars believed that your brain is hardwired at birth and that, perhaps aside from learning some manners, your temperament and behavior are set at the moment of your first breath. Mental disease until the 1930s was generally regarded as the immutable curse of a tainted genetic stock, and to think otherwise smacked of subversion. In the 1950s, Harry Harlow did much to accelerate a change in popular attitudes. He separated a group of infant monkeys from their warm, nurturing mothers and provided cold, mechanical bottle-holding devices in their place. Television viewers were deeply moved by the pathetic result. In sharp contrast to their gregarious, naturally raised siblings, these withdrawn, easily frightened monkeys lived out their lives constantly cowering in the corners of their cages. By the 1960s, it was broadly accepted that severe psychic trauma can leave lasting mental effects, and that experience can indelibly change patterns of behavior, although there were conflicting ideas about how this happens and how those changes might be reversed. Then, too late for Freud to enjoy this confirmation, David Hubel and Torsten Wiesel found evidence that experience not only changes behavior, it physically changes the brain. They found fresh footprints of the environment in a field of synapses.

They stumbled on this bombshell as they were studying ocular dominance columns, the alternating bands of neurons in the visual cortex that receive information exclusively from either the right eye or the left. Covering one eye of a newborn kitten with a translucent membrane to blur its image for a few weeks produced what, in classic laboratory understatement, they called an unexpected effect. Neurons previously connected with the covered eye had actually severed those connections and formed new synapses with cells signaling from the unobstructed eye. Experience had changed the physical structure of the neuron.

Hubel and Wiesel were even more shocked when they looked at the neurons in the thalamus (specifically the LGN), which were carrying signals from the occluded eye to the cortex. Those neurons not only lost their connection with the visual cortex, they became shrunken and pale. Photographs of these dead and dying neurons in the thalamus stunned the scientific community. Here was permanent, destructive, physical change induced not by surgery or by physical trauma, but by sensory deprivation alone. This was graphic evidence that the brain is not completely hardwired at birth, but is molded in a very real sense by personal experience.

During a critical period in early life, there is a fierce competition among the neurons in the thalamus, the relay station for sensory stimuli, to form lasting neural connections in the cortex. The currency in this competition is the transmission of clear signals. Cortical neurons receiving signals from the kitten's covered eye were not content with fuzzy reports of a blurred image. They severed their connections with the bearers of those garbled messages and synapsed instead with axons that carried more interesting signals from the other eye.

During early life, the neurons of the visual cortex are able to disobey their original marching orders, to change their connections and synapse instead, with the highest bidder. The axon reporting about the sharpest contrasts wins this competition. This *plasticity* of the visual cortex, its ability to sever fuzzy connections and establish new ones that are static-free, is lost after kittens are a few months old but in humans it remains for about ten years. The treatment of children with cataract, strabismus, or other causes of early loss of vision in one eye often includes patching the good eye. This is not done to force the bad eye to work harder. It is a kind of therapeutic, affirmative action program designed to make up for a previous, competitive disadvantage. Patching the good eye simply provides an opportunity for signals from the previously handicapped eye to rebuild neural connections to the visual cortex. Without this opportunity to reestablish cortical connections, an eye that has been restored to health will still not see. The younger the patient the greater the benefit of patching will be, and some connections can still be restored until the age of nine or ten.

Sensory stimulation is the young brain's food. Just as visual input shapes the wiring of the visual cortex, early stimulation from the ears builds neural pathways in the auditory cortex. Without proper auditory input, these connections become scrambled and cortical neurons fail to form the neat columns required to process language. Without this necessary neural scaffold, learning to speak becomes a nearly impossible task. If deafness is not diagnosed in the first months of life, normal patterns of speech may be impossible to learn even if hearing is later restored. The necessary cortical connections will simply not be there to do the job. But auditory input also shapes the brain in more subtle ways.

Adults raised in Japan, even those who have learned to speak English very well, are unable to hear any difference at all between the sounds of the letters *r* and *l*. No matter how carefully one enunciates them, the words *rake* and *lake* are indistinguishable. Yet, until the age of about one year, Japanese infants distinguish the *r* and *l* as separate sounds quite easily. After several repetitions of the word *rake,* six- and ten-month-old Japanese babies will grow bored and ignore the speaker, but they respond as if to a new stimulus when the word *lake* is interjected in the series. After one year of age, once they begin to babble, babies growing up in Japan are no longer able to make that distinction nor can they produce the separate sounds of *r* and *l*. They have learned that the adults around them will not hear the difference and their brains are quite literally wired to treat those two sounds as the same. In their first twelve months of life, babies the world over are able to readily distinguish an *r* from an *l,* they can hear the subtle differences in the Spanish sounds for *b, p* and *v,* and they can easily recognize the distinction between the French *u* as in *rue* and *ou* as in *vous*. However, by the time a baby begins to babble, the language she has been listening to has shaped her brain into that of a provincial rather than a global citizen.

Soft bonnets fitted with electrodes were placed on babies to record event-related potentials (ERPs) as they listened to typical sounds of various languages. Infants younger than ten months reacted similarly to their native language and to foreign ones. A few months later, these same babies showed unique patterns of brain activity in their left hemispheres only when they heard sounds typical of their own language.[4] The language a baby hears in the first year of life shapes the neural connections in Wernike's area for language recognition in the left temporal lobe and in Broca's area for speech in the left frontal lobe. Those connections, in turn, determine how it will hear and speak. By the age of ten or twelve months, Chinese babies prattle with the rapid pitch changes unique to their culture, a French boy produces a nasal *n* at the end of *non,* and an African girl easily masters the clicking sound of her native language.[5]

The brain of a small child is an incredible learning machine. Metabolizing glucose much more rapidly than your brain does, it sprouts new synapses at an astonishing rate. A single neuron in the cerebral cortex of a newborn infant has an average of 2,500 synapses. By about the age of twelve, this number has increased to an amazing 15,000 synapses per neuron.[6] Imagine having to answer the phone in an office with that many lines. Only those synapses that repeatedly receive clear and important messages thrive and survive, while those that transmit less riveting information whither and die. Like prize blooms on a rose bush, or marketable apples in an orchard, the number of synapses that reach full fruition reflects a balance between unbridled, unproductive growth and selective pruning.

Out of a lush overgrowth of synapses, only those cultivated by repetition will survive to form clear connections in the developed brain. Repeated sensory stimuli determine which synapses will survive and, in doing so, they stamp the customs and taboos of one's culture in place as if by a branding iron. Familiar sounds, sights, smells, facial expressions, voice inflections, dialect, rituals, cuisine, behavioral norms, all of these make a permanent, physical imprint. Michael Leon at the University of Southern California showed that indelible networks form in a newborn's brain within seconds of the first time it smells its mother's body. The unpredictable events of your early years strengthened the synaptic connections necessary for your survival and deeply etched your likes, dislikes, expectations, prohibitions, pride, and prejudices into the wiring of your young brain. This remarkable plasticity gives children who are born on opposite sides of the globe the marvelous feeling of being at home with the particular languages, foods, and behaviors of the groups in which they happen to find themselves. It also makes them strangers in another culture.

Understanding the surprising role of tactile stimulation in early life has revolutionized the care of premature infants. Those fragile, incubator babies often fail to thrive even though all of their physical needs are carefully met. They have abnormally high levels of stress hormones and a suppressed synthesis of protein. The identical situation was observed in newborn rats raised separately from their mothers. This process was completely reversed with the unlikely treatment of stimulating them with wet paintbrushes to mimic their mothers' licking. When premature infants were taken out of their incubators to be held, touched, and have their backs rubbed, they doubled their rate of weight gain, their stress hormones and protein synthesis returned to normal and they left the hospital much earlier than those not receiving this stimulation. Standard hospital care of premature infants now includes regularly removing them from their incubators to be held, cuddled and massaged.[7]

The physical plasticity of the brain, the ability of sensory input to strengthen synaptic connections, is central to the care of stroke patients and determines the amount of function that they will recover. When a blood clot or a small hemorrhage cuts off the blood flow to a small area of the brain, this *infarct* kills a very circumscribed population of neurons. However, the severity of a stroke is compounded because the neurons surrounding the infarct also stop functioning simply because they are deprived of their customary stimulation from their now-dead neighbors. Even though these cells still have an adequate blood supply, they will also die within a few months unless they can form new neural attachments. They will die of boredom! There is a good reason that physical therapy for stroke patients includes the same kind of exaggerated encouragement and repetition typically lavished on an infant taking its first steps. Just as they were in their infancy, the neurons surrounding the area of a stroke will be pruned unless they are able to form new connections with axons transmitting clear signals forcefully and often. Once again, they will synapse with the highest bidder and their tentative, new connections will be strengthened by repetitive stimulation. It has recently been shown that a small dose of amphetamine, which increases the brain's output of noradrenaline, markedly accelerates this process.[8] Patients who are left to mend on their own after a stroke fare much worse than those who are given small doses of amphetamine and large doses of repetitive training coupled with the same, wide-eyed, overly enthusiastic praise and encouragement that is usually reserved for toddlers.

During the last ten years, a number of studies have confirmed that encouragement and approval continue to facilitate the development of new synapses throughout life and it appears that the more you learn, the more synapses you develop. Autopsy studies performed at the University of California at Los Angeles showed that college graduates who remained mentally active throughout their adult life had 40 percent more synapses in their brains than high school dropouts and they also had more synapses than college graduates who did not remain mentally active in later life. Indeed, there is growing evidence that education may serve as a deterrent to Alzheimer's disease.[9]

Something else happens to your brain as you age. Remember the NMDA receptor in the hippocampus and how it responds only to separate signals arriving simultaneously? Dr. Tsien at his memory laboratory at Princeton University has discovered that until about the age of puberty, it will respond only to signals that arrive less than 250 thousandths of a second apart. At about the age of twelve, that interval narrows to only 150 one-thousandths of a second. The effect of narrowing that window is to markedly reduce your capacity to remember and to learn. Dr. Tsien, the only child in his rural Chinese village to be accepted to a college, came to this country as a young graduate student. He is fond of saying that if he had come here ten years sooner, before this receptor change occurred, he would now be able to speak without a foreign accent. In fact, age twelve seems to be the upper limit at which learning a second language comes easily.

For these two reasons—the longer time interval during which the NMDA receptor can respond, and the incredible proliferation of young synapses—it is in the first months and years of life that the most profound imprints of experience are stamped on the brain.

As sociologists, psychologists, and psychiatrists have long claimed in a figurative sense, we now know that the early years are, quite literally, formative. Laboratory rats developed and retained fully one-fourth more synapses when William Greenough at the University of Illinois exposed them to an environment enriched with toys, food, exercise devices, and playmates. This physical change within their brains was mirrored in a corresponding change in these animals' behavior. They performed better in mazes and with other tests of learning ability when compared to other rats raised in standard, drab cages.

Craig Ramey, at the University of Alabama, exposed a group of impoverished inner-city children as young as six weeks to an enriched environment with active learning, good nutrition, toys, and playmates. After twelve years, IQ testing and PET scans to measure their brain activity showed significant gains when they were compared to a control group of similar children who did not benefit from that early intervention. Perhaps the most stunning difference after twelve years was that only 13 percent of the intervention group had failed a grade or more, compared with 50 percent of the control group.

These findings do not mean that buying the right toys for your baby and playing tapes of Mozart near her crib will increase her later chances of admission to Harvard. It is not the price of the paraphernalia in the nursery that matters, but the quality of the human interaction that takes place there. For the toddler as well as for stroke victims, smiles, enthusiasm, and loving encouragement establish and cultivate new synapses. The brain needs to see a happy face and to hear occasional laughter to cement its neural circuitry. The encouraging sounds of "Yes! Good! That's it!" help to mark a synapse for preservation rather than for pruning. Even when stodgy old professors learn something new, they can be heard to reward themselves with a gleeful "Aha!" Celebrating a new discovery increases the likelihood that it will be remembered.

Learning how experiences physically mold the inherited shape of the brain has turned the old nature-versus-nurture debate on its ear. Heredity and the environment do not work separately, but hand in glove. Stress; success; failure; the relative richness or impoverishment of the environment; the nature of interpersonal relationships; all of these invisible forces cause molecular changes—and the hereditary material in the nucleus of the neuron is programmed to respond to these changes. Bits of DNA lie dormant, waiting for the right inducement to replicate a specific molecule of protein, and that inducement often comes from the environment.

Schizophrenia is a good example of the interaction of nature and nurture. The fact that heredity plays a role in schizophrenia is clear. Only 1 percent of the general population develops this disease. However, 6 percent of the parents of schizophrenics, 9 percent of their siblings, 17 percent of their fraternal twins, and 48 percent of their identical twins also show signs of schizophrenia.[10] If heredity were not a factor, there would be no reason to expect a lower incidence of schizophrenia among fraternal twins than among identical twins. But if a genetic defect causes schizophrenia, and identical twins have identical DNA, why are only 48 percent rather than 100 percent of them affected? The answer is that this genetic abnormality alone is not sufficient to cause the disease. An abnormal gene is merely a faulty switch that can be turned on by a stimulus that might otherwise have no ill effect. Subtle, perhaps even commonplace factors in the environment may cause those faulty genes to express themselves and produce the perplexing behavioral and perceptual distortions characteristic of that illness. Those factors are common enough to trip the faulty gene in 48 percent of the identical twins who carry it.

Fifteen pairs of identical twins in which one twin was schizophrenic and the other was not were examined with magnetic resonance imaging. In twelve of these pairs, the scan of the twin with the disease showed shrinking of brain tissue surrounding the ventricles.[11] Each twin had a susceptible gene, but in only one of them did some necessary environmental factor or factors trip the switch and produce an abnormal molecule or molecules. Both nature and nurture altered the structure of the brain and distorted its behavior. It is impossible to view the effects of one in isolation from the other.

Every young brain responds to its environment. Its growth is stunted when its necessary diet of nurturing stimuli is stolen by neglect or poisoned by abuse, and its huge potential can be unfettered without waiting for pharmaceutical or technological advances. Nothing more complicated than consistent, kind, personal attention holds the promise of enormous rewards for the individual child as well as for society. The absence of this early, reliable, basic nurturing has a tragic cost. This knowledge has already inspired many new social programs for child care and education. But for many, even such successful programs as Head Start are far too little and probably much too late.

A harvest of discontent grows from seeds sown during the first three years of life and, once planted, often leaves a bitter legacy, a cycle of violence and abuse that is passed from one generation to the next. Frequently, we turn off the evening news numbed by the report of a senseless outrage. An unremarkable child commits a cold-blooded murder. A slighted employee turns an assault weapon on co-workers and then himself. A remorseless suspect is arraigned for a series of unprovoked, heinous crimes and we begin to search for evidence of faulty wiring in the past of the perpetrator.

All of the evidence suggests that axons begin to make their fateful synapses during the critical, first three years of life.[12] Our challenge is to unravel the remaining mysteries of this early wiring of the brain, to learn which molecular maladies and which critical events in the early spring of the neuron cause its young vines to grow twisted and to bear such bitter fruit. Answering this challenge may finally lead us to be proper stewards of this amazing garden of good and evil.

9

Beyond the Yellow Brick Road

The Brain Is a Supercomputer and Much, Much More

IT WOULD HAVE BEEN LOVELY—and it probably would have confirmed your intuitive feelings about the operation of your brain—if all of the reports of the visual cortex converged toward a single place, a mission control center that monitors all incoming sensory signals and responds with the neural equivalent of "All systems are go for launch!"—or perhaps only for lunch. But the paths of the yellow brick road do not converge toward one point. Signals branch out from the visual cortex in all directions at once, and I can imagine Hubel and Wiesel parroting the famous Laurel and Hardy line, "Now this is a *fine* mess you've gotten us into!" It is a tribute to the patience and ingenuity of neuroanatomists that we can follow these pathways at all, and it is precisely because visual signals travel so widely that we have learned how the brain is organized. Following the faint signals from the eye provides an unparalleled view of the brain. From the visual cortex, these signals travel to a surprisingly large number of areas in the brain concerned not only with what you see, but with where you look. On the day you were born, you began to explore your amorphous surroundings from the mattress of your crib as though the entire world was simply an extended part of you. When you started to move around on your own two feet, and you began to feel separate from that external world, you started to build bridges across a perplexing gulf by pointing, touching, talking, and thinking about the interface between you and everything else. That construction project continues today and your eye movements are essential to it.

The owl needs to swivel its head to look from one place to another because its eyes are fixed in their sockets. You are spared that inconvenience by having eyes that rotate quite freely by means of twelve muscles, six attached to each eye. Reading these words involves an intricately choreographed ballet. Pairs of muscles on opposite sides of each eye move them smoothly and precisely from one word to the next with no overshoot, while the other eight muscles maintain exactly the right tension to control upward or downward drift. Any misstep produces disabling double vision. The marionettelike movements of your twelve ocular muscles occur at the behest of two puppeteers simultaneously. While they are under the voluntary control of the motor cortex in your frontal lobe, they are at the same time the involuntary servants of your vestibular apparatus. This internal gyroscope in the bones behind your ear evolved from the ancient arrangement of a grain of sand embedded near sensitive hairs of jellyfish and sea anemones. Now, this gravity detector drives your sense of balance and sends signals to neurons in your brain stem that control eye movements, which are completely involuntary.

You maintain a very steady view of the world from a sometimes wildly moving vantage point because of neural signals arriving from sensory hairs and shifting granules of calcium

149

in the semicircular canals of your inner ear as well as from all eight lobes of your cortex, your cerebellum, your midbrain, and your brain stem. These signals finally converge onto neurons on each side of your brain stem that keep your eyes on target as your head bobs and weaves its way through the world. If your eyes did not compensate for your body's motion with movements of their own, you would need to stop every few steps and steady your head to see where you were going. When you suddenly spin your head to the right, your vestibular reflex turns your eyes to the left with the same speed and to the same degree, so that your view of the world remains undisturbed. Because of your vestibular reflex, you can keep your eye on a fly ball as you run to catch it, even if you trip and fall in the attempt.

Your satellite dish for the photon is mounted on an ingenious tracking system. While most of its signals are building a visual universe within your brain, others are responding to your internal gyroscope, keeping you upright, oriented, and on a steady course. It not only keeps your eye on the ball, it keeps *you* "on the ball" as well. Precise reports of your eye movements are relayed to your hands and arms and tell them where to reach. Signals generated by your eye movements tell your head when to duck and your torso which way to turn as you maneuver through the world, and they convey this critical information without your giving it a thought. They are a critical link to the outside world.

As you look around the room, your eyes do not sweep across the scene as smoothly as you might imagine. You see the world one section at a time. Only one small area is focused at your fovea, that small area at the center of your retina with its dense concentration of cones. The one or two words that your foveae are aiming at now are in sharp focus while the rest of the page is poorly resolved. As you aim your foveae toward one area of interest after another, your eyes move in extremely quick jerks called saccades—from the French word for jolt. You do not see a blur during these eye movements because they last less than the one-twentieth of a second required for an image to reach your awareness.

Looking at the Mona Lisa is a ballet choreographed jointly by your brain and the features of the painting. Your eyes are inexorably drawn to Mona Lisa's face and stop briefly at each of her eyes. You remember this snapshot as your eyes move to other areas of interest, which da Vinci has strategically placed throughout the painting to make them do just that. Your view of the painting is your memory of all of the snapshots your brain has taken during the brief pauses between saccades.

Only when you track something moving across your field of vision do your eyes move smoothly. The image of a solidly hit ball sailing over the center field fence is kept on the same area of the retina throughout your tracking movement and, as you look out from the window of a moving train, it is impossible to keep your eyes still. As if magnetized, your eyes will lock on to some feature moving by, perhaps a telephone pole, and follow its movement smoothly until it passes. They will then make a completely involuntary, quick saccade toward the front of the train, during which you see nothing, to pick up the next telephone pole, house, or cow and smoothly follow it backward again, an involuntary, repetitive movement called nystagmus.

Moving a pattern of vertical stripes across your field of vision will produce the same unwilled eye movements. Before the advent of computerized axial tomography and magnetic resonance imaging, this simple technique was often used to test the integrity of the brain stem and to determine the location of lesions affecting the ocular motor pathways. If neural fibers coming to the brain stem from the right parietal lobe are damaged, nystagmus will be induced by moving the stripes to the left, as is normal, but the patient's eyes will remain still when the stripes are moved to the right. The reverse is true if the pathways from the left parietal lobe are damaged. If the eyes remain stationary while stripes move across the visual field in both directions, this is an ominous sign of brain stem damage. In this grave condition, reflex eye movements are paralyzed even though the patient can still, voluntarily, move his eyes in all directions at the behest of the frontal cortex.

Normally, your eyes, hands, and body are constantly exchanging information about their relative positions. Signals reporting about your eye movements will help you turn this page and they will cause you to adjust your step in mid-stride thoughtlessly and automatically when you suddenly approach a step or a curb. This is possible because many branches of the yellow brick road are two-way streets. Neurons at each end keep track of the activity at the other, with signals constantly traveling in both directions. If you have ever watched a movie in 3-D, I-Max, or Cinerama, you have probably moved involuntarily in your seat as you appeared to be rushing toward the lip of the Grand Canyon or hurtling around a bend on a roller coaster. Your body was responding to something called *visual flow.*

As you look forward from the front of a subway train, the end of the tunnel stays in the center of your field of view as you approach it, while the walls appear to get larger and move outward as you pass. This predictable sense of visual flow enables you to navigate successfully as you walk down the street, around a corner, and up the stairs. It helps you keep your car in its proper lane, and a highly developed sense of visual flow is essential if you want to qualify as a fighter pilot. This sense is impaired in Alzheimer's disease. Early in their disease, elderly patients get lost in familiar neighborhoods, not because of a loss of memory or vision, but because they lose the feedback between their retinal image and their motor pathways. Even when their vision and memory are still reasonably well-preserved, loss of the sense of visual flow impairs their ability to know whether they are moving straight ahead or going in circles. When you are in a fog or in unfamiliar surroundings, the connection of your eyes to your vestibular and motor pathways can keep you moving successfully through even the most dimly seen or poorly understood environs.

But the main business of the neural pathways coming from the visual cortex is to piece together a thousand fragments, to attach memories and meaning to sketchy signals, and to interpret what you see. To do this, signals from the visual cortex pass through several areas of the brain, which appear to play a version of the game twenty questions. Each of these areas seems to ask one question and, as each question is answered, important new threads are woven into the rich fabric of cognition. We have learned about these areas because of the peculiar symptoms that result when they are injured. For example:

1. An area in the temporal lobe appears to ask the question, "Have I seen this before?" The cells in this region respond only if they can match an image with a memory. Injury here results in agnosia, the perplexing inability to recognize a previously familiar object. Patients suffering from agnosia look at a key a moment after being told what it is, and simply do not recognize or "know it again." The shape, size, color, and visual texture are no longer sufficient to identify it.

2. When an object disappears from view, the cells in one region of the frontal lobe seem to ask, "Where was it?" and they remember. The neurons in this area told you which drawer to open to find your socks this morning. An injury here causes a form of visual memory loss that makes hide-and-seek a hopeless game. It produces the curious inability to find an object even moments after

watching where it was hidden. A baby will enjoy the game peek-a-boo only after about one year of age, when the synapses in this part of the frontal lobe have developed. Prior to that, the game is ignored because an object lost from sight is lost from memory as well.

3. A particularly versatile group of cells in the parietal lobe asks, "Can I reach it?" Injury to this area causes a divorce of the visual world from the tactile world and makes turning a page a hit-or-miss proposition. Remarkably, a single neuron in this area receives information from nearly every part of the brain.

- From signals sent by the *frontal lobe* and *midbrain,* it registers the position of your eye muscles and then calculates the position of the object relative to you.
- From signals sent by the somatic sensory cortex in the *parietal lobe,* it registers the location of your arms and hands in space.
- With signals from the visual cortex in the *occipital lobe,* it registers the location of the object of your attention in your visual field.
- From the *midbrain,* it even registers your level of interest and emotional investment in the object of regard.

After evaluating all of this information, these virtuoso cells in your parietal lobe direct neurons in your frontal lobe, your cerebellum, and your midbrain to choreograph the precise movements required to turn a page, to catch a baseball, or to deflect a snowball. This is a far cry from the simple task of the ganglion cell. There, according to rules laid down by evolution, only one condition needs to be met for the ganglion cell to fire, a difference in the degree of stimulation in the two parts of its tiny, circular receptive field. The receptive field of these remark-

able neurons in the parietal lobe is a network spread throughout the brain and the rules that govern their responses are too
complex to be clearly stated. In milliseconds, they must differentiate a threat from a treat. In an instant they will decide
whether you will reach out an open hand, raise a clenched fist,
or prepare to duck and cover. Those important rules are written less by evolution than by your personal training.

Until the mid 1970s, it was believed that the brain is organized in a steplike arrangement of progressively more sophisticated centers. It certainly appears that after the ganglion cell
asks "Is there a contrasting border?" neurons in the cortex then
ask about motion, color, form, and depth and relay the answers
to higher centers of the brain that ask specific questions in
turn, such as: "What is this?" "Where have I seen it before?"
"Can I reach it?" "What does it feel like?" "Has it changed?"
"Does it remind me of something?" "Does it change the way I
feel?" "Am I going to do something about it?" Naturally, no
such time-consuming questions are consciously thought out.
They are asked and answered in an instant by neurons
responding to a set of signals so specific that they seem to be
constantly asking a single question, different from and more
complex than the one asked in the preceding center.

The notion of a hierarchy of centers, each more complex than
the previous, implied that there should be a highest center at
which the most complete representation and understanding of
a perception occurs, the central processor we all seem to feel is
operating somewhere behind our eyes. Prior to 1980, the problem for neuroscience was that no such center, nor even any reasonable candidates for such a center, could be found. The yellow
brick road seemed instead to branch endlessly in a hopeless
maze, and the organization of the brain remained a mystery.

Major steps in understanding often come from examining
small bits of information that seem not to fit. Semir Zeki,

professor of neurobiology at the University of London, did just that. He refused to dismiss occasional, puzzling reports that kept cropping up in the neurological literature. Patients with injuries to the visual cortex would occasionally report only a loss of color vision. Based on the current understanding of the brain, these injuries should have also produced at least small areas of blindness, but they did not. Because these cases were rare, the discrepancy was attributed to insufficient testing and these reports were dismissed as insignificant.

Dr. Zeki saw their significance. By pursuing this inconsistency—cortical injuries producing loss of color vision with no loss of formed vision—he was able to prove that perception does *not* proceed in sequential, serial steps. He discovered that the neat columns of neurons in the main area of the visual cortex extract detailed information only about form, and they immediately delegate to adjacent cortical areas the more specialized tasks of appreciating color, motion, and depth perception. Rather than one visual cortex, there are several, each specialized for a specific function, each built to simultaneously extract one of these essential features of vision from the signals of the ganglion cell.

Injury to one of these areas accounted for a complete loss of color vision with no detectable blind spot. More recently, patients have been studied whose injuries involved only the area required to detect motion. This produces the bizarre condition of being unable to perceive the continuous movement of an object from one place to another. The effect is like watching a movie from which sections have been removed. For these patients, a car approaching in the distance suddenly appears nearby without any perceived transition. Crossing the street takes on new terrors. Dr. Zeki showed that each of these nearby cortical areas has its own topographical map of the visual world and each has its own very specialized machinery for extracting

156

an essential feature of visual perception. And—here is the important point—all of these parallel systems perform their tasks simultaneously. In computer jargon, this would be called parallel circuitry.

As computers began to influence our culture, they also impacted our thinking about the brain. A standard personal computer processes bits of information in a serial fashion, one after the other and each in a matter of microseconds. Neural circuits operate in milliseconds, one thousand times more slowly. The brain makes up for this relatively slow speed by allowing information to travel along parallel neural circuits simultaneously. It saves time the way you do when you slice string beans bunched side by side rather than one at a time. The greater the number of beans you can align, the greater the efficiency, and if there is one outstanding feature of your brain, it is the huge number of its neurons.

Billions of neurons in the cerebral cortex are arranged in six parallel layers and in millions of individual columns. This is precisely what computer engineers dream about, a massive, multilayered, parallel-distributed processor. Dr. Zeki showed that the visual cortex, like a parallel processor, divides large jobs into smaller tasks, dedicates each to its own work space and processes all of them simultaneously. Computers were subsequently built incorporating this parallel circuitry. These machines do not simply respond to preprogrammed instructions; they learn and adapt on their own, and in the next chapter we will see how they work. However, no manmade computer can truly mimic the brain because no microcircuit even comes close to the complexity of the neuron. Edwin Land, of the Polaroid Corporation, discovered an element of this complexity when, in 1983, he learned an amazing thing about the way you see colors.

At the age of seventeen, while Land was a freshman at

Harvard, he became interested in polarized light. He took a two-year leave of absence and, with a small group of young scientists, founded a laboratory not far from the campus. In 1937, this became the Polaroid Corporation, which soon was heavily involved in research for the military. In the late 1940s, with the introduction of the Polaroid Land Camera, Land became a very rich man, but he never lost his keen enthusiasm for basic science. At the age of seventy-four, one year after he stepped down as head of the Polaroid Corporation, he solved a riddle he had been working on for most of his adult life, one that had been puzzling scientists for centuries. He fit one more piece into the parallel puzzles of light and the neuron.

Ever since Newton first explained the rainbow of colors seen when white light passes through a prism and is separated into bands of different wavelengths, we have been taught that an object looks red simply because it reflects long-wave or red light, and absorbs the rest. The uncomfortable truth is that when an object is moved from direct sunlight into the shade—or into a room lit by fluorescent light—the wavelength of its reflected light changes so dramatically that its color should change as well. Yet, in defiance of physical laws, a red object continues to look red to a human observer under each of those varied lighting conditions. The inescapable but troubling conclusion is that objects are not endowed with codes or labels that can be analyzed passively as colors. This is referred to as the paradox of "color inconstancy."

Darwin pointed out that this is not a trivial problem. Color is more than just the frivolous makeup of Mother Nature. The survival of many species depends on their ability to appreciate color in order to identify ripe fruit, to avoid poisonous berries, to recognize the markings of predators and prey and to appreciate the sexual display of a mate. They—and we—must have a mechanism to actively construct a constant color from the changing wavelengths reflecting from an object's surface.

Edwin Land described the difficult task that the brain would need to perform in order to construct a color that remains constant in sun and shade: "It would need to analyze the changing wavelengths of the light reflected from an object *and continuously compare those with the wavelengths simultaneously reflected from the surfaces which surround it*" (italics added).[1]

Semir Zeki found an area of the occipital lobe that performs precisely this kind of analysis. Its neurons have color-sensitive receptive fields that can be of any size. These neurons form separate, flexible topographical maps upon which they compare the wavelength composition of objects both large and small with the wavelengths that surround them. Although you may have never had an advanced math class and probably have never considered the intellectual paradox of color inconstancy, a tiny area at the back of your brain is solving this problem with the following bit of calculus. Reading the next paragraph is completely optional, but remember: Although you may have no flair for mathematics, your neurons perform this bit of calculation instantly, every time you shift your gaze!

Here goes! The ratio of the intensity of light of a given wavelength reflected from a surface (the numerator) and the average intensity of light of the same wavelength reflected by its surrounding surfaces (the denominator) is determined. The logarithm of this ratio is taken. These calculations are repeated for each of the three wavebands: short (blue), medium (green), and long (red), which are absorbed by the three kinds of cones in your retina. The results, plotted on three axes, give a remarkably accurate prediction of the color of the surface *regardless* of the intensity of the light reflected from it.[2]

Red remains red, indoors or out. Color is the product of the brain's calculation and not of an object's surface. The best we can do to define a rich, ruby red, aside from saying "Here, look!" is with a three-dimensional, logarithmic plot. This is a bit like describing a symphony by reporting about the movements on the stage, the notes in the written score, and the squiggles of an oscilloscope attached to a microphone. It is so much more satisfying, though less objective, to simply say, "Here, listen!" Our appreciation of the sounds and sights of the world requires both the parallel circuitry of a computer whose fluid complexity we have yet to understand and the unparalleled brilliance of the individual neuron.

THIS BRINGS US TO a major focus of contemporary neuroscience, *the binding problem*. How does your brain form a seamlessly unified, three-dimensional perception from scattered fragments. At the same instant that the visual attributes of an object are assembled in several parts of your occipital cortex, the sounds associated with it are formed in your temporal lobe. The smells, ideas, and emotions attached to it are produced in still other, widely scattered areas throughout your brain. Somehow, your brain "binds" separate bits of color, sound and emotion into useful, unified, multisensate perceptions. From these, it creates a world in which you are both an observer and integral part.

As early as 1949, Donald O. Hebb at McGill University in Montreal suggested how this might occur in his seminal book, *The Organization of Behavior*.[3] It is often said that timing is everything, and Hebb proposed that the timing of the neuron's signals is indeed the key to binding separate fragments of their electrochemical buzz into meaningful perceptions and useful behavior. After earning a Ph.D. in psychology at Harvard University in 1936, Hebb returned to Canada, where he was born and raised, and accepted a teaching position at McGill University. Purely on theoretical grounds, he proposed that the glue that binds together a single perception is the *synchronous firing* of participating neurons.[4] His brilliant theories gained attention only later, when the technology to test them was developed. Since his death in 1985, evidence to support them has continued to mount. Within the last few years, simultaneous, multichannel microelectrode recordings from large arrays of neurons have shown unmistakably that he was right.[5] Neurons collaborate like instrumentalists playing in separate sections of an orchestra. When they act in precisely timed concert, their signals coalesce into a single, coherent piece of music.

The sight of a loaf of fresh bread leaving the oven and its distinct aroma are "bound" together by the coordinated timing and simultaneous activity of neurons in the olfactory cortex near the front of the brain and in the visual cortex at the back. The synchronous firing of their signals at forty spikes per second (40 Hz) is what binds together the sight of the bread, its fresh-baked aroma and perhaps, in another area of the cortex, an extraneous childhood memory of your mother's kitchen. The result is a single, *experienced* perception.

For Francis Crick and for Christof Koch who works with him at the Salk Institute, this idea, coupled with more recent experimental findings, raised the question of attention, or awareness. Of the countless distracting and competing perceptions presented to it, how does your brain focus, or tune in, on a particular object of interest? How are you able to follow a single conversation amid the din of a crowded cocktail party or read the hands of a small clock on a cluttered shelf across the room? Crick is the British physicist and biochemist who shared the 1962 Nobel Prize with James Watson for discovering the structure of the DNA molecule. He is now Distinguished Research Professor at the Salk Institute in La Jolla, California, and one of the world's foremost theoretical neuroscientists. In 1994, Drs. Crick and Koch postulated that the synchronous firing of neurons in the thalamus, the sensory gateway to the cortex, might be responsible for this critical ability to zero in on a specific set of stimuli. The thalamus is not only a relay station, it is a rigorous checkpoint where arriving sensory signals are carefully sorted, checked, and very selectively relayed to appropriate cortical areas to compete for your conscious awareness.[6]

Thalamic neurons have been observed to fire, not only at similar rates of about 40 Hz, but in a remarkably coordinated pattern called gamma oscillation. They fire precisely in rhythm and on the beat like drummers in a parade. Crick and Koch liken the thalamus to a conductor using these oscillating signals as a baton to direct relevant sets of cortical neurons with its rhythms. Like a flashlight beam aimed toward the cortex, a stream of these oscillating signals from the thalamus could determine where you direct your attention, what you think about, or what you do. This stream of oscillating signals from the thalamus could be the neural correlate of awareness; the tuning device that determines which words you will hear in a crowded room, whether the sound of a dripping faucet will keep you awake at night, and how quickly you will respond to your alarm clock in the morning.[7]

As you concentrate on this page, your thalamus may selectively enhance the visual stimuli coming from these words and subdue the unnoticed sounds coming from outside your room, sounds that might otherwise cause you sit bolt upright in the middle of the night. Serious practitioners of meditation speak of the detachment, peace, and rejuvenation that come from shrinking one's attention to nothing but the thought of a single sound.[8] The Crick-Koch theory suggests that this could be the result of severely narrowing the beam of oscillations from the thalamus. Directing these signals to only one tiny area of the cortex and leaving the rest totally devoid of sensory input—literally disconnected from the outside world—could produce just the kind of rare silence of the mind that is achieved during deep meditation. A disciplined, meditative focus is what differentiates this unique state from the unregulated hallucinations that occur during prolonged sensory deprivation.

At the 1999 annual meeting of the Society for Neuroscience, Dr. Rudolfo Llinás presented his findings on a similar, yet even more far-reaching theory. Dr. Llinás is professor and chairman of the department of physiology and neuroscience at New York University Medical School, chief editor of the journal *Neuroscience,* and chairman of NASA's neuroscience division. His research, like that of Crick and Koch, suggests that the thalamus is much more than a relay station sending sensory signals to the cerebral cortex. There is a surprisingly complex traffic pattern along this pathway. It appears that far more signals flow down from the cortex than come up from the thalamus. In addition to sensation, the traffic on those pathways influences muscle movement, emotions, and complex thought. Dr. Llinás proposed that the signals coming down from the cortex to the thalamus serve as traffic directors. They select the signals that the cortex is most anxious to receive and expedite their trip. It is in these thalamo-cortical pathways, he suggests, that your brain begins to organize random signals into complete perceptions, actions, thoughts, movements, and even consciousness itself.[9] This is where you start to fabricate your world and your behavior.

A dramatic new treatment for Parkinson's disease—and for patients suffering from severe depression—provides additional evidence that the thalamus is much more than a gateway to the sensory cortex. The oscillating, highly organized signals traveling between the thalamus and the cortex were discovered to be abnormal in these patients—whose problems had more to do with movement and mood than with sensory issues. An attempt was made to relieve their symptoms by surgically implanting electrodes in this area and stimulating it in the same way that pacemakers are used to regulate the heart. Given the precise nature of the surgery involved, it is remarkable that this experimental procedure could be done at all. Even more remarkable is the fact that it has produced some dramatic improvements.

Abnormal thalamo-cortical signals have been found in a variety of brain diseases, all of which share a strange connection. They have in common several unexplained symptoms such as hand wringing, deep sadness, ringing in the ears, unrelenting tremors, muscle rigidity, spasms, or choreoform movements. These uncontrolled, dancelike or writhing movements are seen in Huntington's chorea and many other diseases, including the series of disorders that share the name cerebral palsy. The oscillating signals of the thalamus are abnormal in all of these diseases. Llinás found that when thalamic signals oscillate at a rapid rate, the brain is awake and alert and behavior is focused and efficient. When those oscillations slow down, important parts of the cortex become unregulated. In a motor area, this loss of thalamic regulation can cause rigidity, tremor, or uncontrolled hand wringing. Similar deregulation of the auditory cortex results in disturbing tinnitus, or ringing in the ears. An unregulated prefrontal cortex leads to profound sadness. At last, there is a single explanation for a baffling and bizarre group of symptoms suffered in a number of seemingly unrelated neurologic disease.

Electroshock therapy, popular a generation ago, was a sledgehammer approach to the problem of depression and psychosis.

Llinás has suggested that the suffering caused by a wide variety of neurologic disorders might be ended by restoring normal oscillation patterns in the thalamo-cortical pathways with precise, pinpoint applications of electric, pacemaker-like stimuli. Understanding the timing of the neuron's signals is far more important than Dr. Hebb could have imagined in 1949—and this story gets even better.

10

The Shape of an Idea

Neuronal Ensembles

DR. HEBB WENT ON TO SUGGEST that the neuron learns from experience. Since this may be the most important concept in contemporary neuroscience, I will rephrase it more precisely. The *timing* of the electrochemical events at the synapse can change the subsequent *behavior* of that synapse. If an axon fires *repeatedly,* its synapses will become *more efficient* at causing its neighbor to fire. Suddenly, the neuron was given credit for some intelligence. Hebb proposed that the neuron remembers what came before and that it alters its response accordingly. This was purely a guess in 1949, but it was the pivot upon which the rest of his theories in *The Organization of Behavior* turned. Happily, Hebb lived to see his theory confirmed in the laboratory. Exactly as he had predicted, the frequent firing of an axon *does* strengthen its synapses. When an impulse arrives at a synapse while calcium levels are still elevated from a previous firing, a buildup of calcium occurs, which releases a larger amount of transmitter from the synaptic vesicles and produces a measurably stronger signal. This may sound like a small, even trivial, matter. In fact, it is evidence of a natural rather than a supernatural source of your mental capacity. It is the biological basis for your ability to remember, to learn, and to behave intelligently.

Hebb's novel idea of a synapse that produces a stronger signal when fired repeatedly has been given a shorthand name, the *Hebbian synapse,* a term that is used as much by computer whizzes as by neurobiologists. It is the essential ingredient in neural network computers, machines that are capable of learning.

An ordinary computer is quite dumb. It amazes you only because it is loaded with lines of code that are installed at the factory and with each software application that you buy. It must be given step-by-step instructions on how to respond to each keystroke or mouse click. The person writing the code must think of everything, because your computer cannot think at all. If you misspell your input slightly or use upper case when the code calls for lower case, your computer will stare at you with an annoyingly unresponsive screen. In 1982, John Hopfield, a molecular biologist turned physicist at Caltech University in Pasadena, developed a new type of computer with an internal design based on the Hebbian synapse.

The Hopfield network, or neural network computer as it came to be known, is loaded with very few coded instructions. It is given a general idea of what success will look like (checkmate = capture the opponent's king) and a few simple rules about how to achieve it (bishops can move only diagonally). Its microcircuits, acting like Hebb's adjustable synapses, become more effective (increasing the weight of their input) with each operation that leads toward success. It gains proficiency the same way that you learn to win friends and influence people, by sticking to a few simple rules learned when you were young (share, cooperate, do unto others . . .), and then, by paying attention to what works and what doesn't. As each microcircuit adjusts its output based on the shifting strengths of its inputs, these computers learned to play chess, recognize faces, and navigate a maze. The speed, efficiency, and capabilities of these computers took a giant leap in 1986, when a group of psychologists at the University of California at San Diego added another brainlike feature to them. Like so many before them, they were struck by the brain's organization as a parallel, distributed processor. They began building computers with several networks rather than one, and they placed these networks in parallel layers, like the sheets of neurons in the retina, cortex, and other key areas of the brain. They started with three layers. The lowest layer, the input layer, was connected to the outside world. In the next hidden layer, each unit was connected to every unit in the input layer. The highest layer, the output layer, was wired with each of its units connected to every unit in the hidden layer.

With this simple plan, Terry Sejnowski and Charles Rosenberg put on a striking demonstration in 1987. A computer that they named NETtalk learned to read and speak English. It learned the same way that you did—by example. It was given no rules of grammar or pronunciation, but only some text and phonetic transcriptions from two training sources. One was an excerpt from Merriam-Webster's Pocket Dictionary and the other was an unusual choice, the unedited speech of a child. NETtalk's output was recorded and played back through a digital speech synthesizer to make the demonstration more lifelike.

At first, NETtalk produced only babble, a confused string of sounds. Gradually, much like a human infant, it learned the distinction between vowels and consonants, began to recognize word boundaries, and then produced strings of pseudo-words. After about ten readings of the input material, this language-learning computer produced intelligible words very similar to the speech of a small child. Later it began to transfer what it had learned from its limited training material and could read words it had never encountered before. Clearly, it was not merely looking up what it had been trained on. It had learned to generalize, to mimic the fuzzy thinking of humans and to deal with probabilities the way we do. Unlike the rigid responses of most machines, parallel distributed neural networks understand "sort of" and "maybe," they draw inferences from similarities, build concepts from sketchy clues and derive generalized conclusions from specific examples.[1] The architecture of these computers, like the microstructure of the brain, correlates directly with their behavior. The remarkable NETtalk demonstration was accomplished by a computer with less than five hundred units and twenty thousand connections. There are about five thousand neurons beneath a patch of your cortex no bigger than the head of a pin, and each of those neurons can have tens of thousands of synapses. And yet, even a computer with a similar number of connections would fall far short of the brain's complexity by ignoring the molecular and biological behavior of the individual neuron.

Hebb is often considered the father of artificial intelligence, but his insights proved even more influential in probing the mystery of human thinking. A neuron's signal can choose among a staggering number of pathways through the brain. Hebb predicted that unlike Robert Frost, a neural impulse will usually choose the path most traveled. He theorized that because some synapses would be strengthened by repeated firing, they would briefly establish preferred, more efficient routes of transmission. Subsequent signals would follow these pathways much as a drop of water will travel more readily down a previously moistened piece of yarn than down a dry one.

Hebb then made the audacious suggestion that the brain would organize itself into temporary *cell assemblies*. The brain, he said, is constantly making subtle changes based on the

169

frequency with which groups of synapses fire. Subsets of several thousands of neurons act as a coordinated ensemble when the connections between them are briefly strengthened by repeated, synchronous firing. Such a group of ephemerally associated neurons might correspond to an image, a phrase, an idea, or a component of a specific behavior.

This notion of neuronal ensembles performing cognitive functions was a brand-new way of thinking about the brain in 1949. Today, it is a cornerstone of brain science. With simultaneous recordings from large numbers of neurons, one can see them forming cell assemblies as their synapses are strengthened by repetitive firing, exactly as Hebb had envisioned on purely theoretical grounds. In laboratories around the world, the focus of research is shifting. More significant than the rigid, anatomical regions of the brain are the changing patterns of association between widely dispersed neurons. Hebb would have enjoyed reading a compilation of recent research by Dr. Geoffrey Schoenbaum. He calls Hebb's ideas "the underpinnings of the investigation of ensemble behavior discussed in this volume,"[2] and he describes the wealth of information coming out of those studies as "exactly what D. O. Hebb described in 1949 when presenting his ideas regarding the organization of cellular activity in the cortex and the resultant emergence of consciousness and motivated activity." Confirmed by a brand-new technology, Hebb's theory is the basis for the current revolution in our understanding of the brain.

Neuronal ensembles or, as Hebb called them, cell assemblies, do not respect the borders of the brain's lobes and they are not restricted to its defined, anatomic regions and pathways. They can span the length and breadth of the brain. They are not fixed, they cannot be pinned down, and they exist only for as long as their member neurons are *simultaneously* and *synchronously* active.

The constant shaping and reshaping of the ephemeral cell assemblies described by Hebb is sometimes referred to as *synaptic plasticity*. This is an unfortunate use of the word *plasticity,* which is usually used in connection with permanent, physical changes in the brain, the growth of new synapses and the death of bypassed neurons that Hubel and Wiesel had discovered by covering one eye of a kitten. Unlike "synaptic plasticity," true, long-lasting plasticity occurs only in the developing brain, or during the first weeks or months after an injury or stroke. It involves anatomical changes in the brain and, once established, those changes are difficult or impossible to reverse. In contrast, the continual, fleeting changes in the shape, size, and location of Hebb's cell assemblies are based solely on the timing of the signals firing at their synapses. Their neurons briefly join in the singing of an electrochemical tune, but they undergo no structural change.

Hebb envisioned that these cell assemblies would overlap, so that any single neuron could belong to several of them. Activating one assembly could then lead to the activation of others, and these fundamental building blocks could quickly organize themselves into more detailed perceptions, more elaborate memories, or more complex behaviors. The fleeting outline of a neuronal ensemble is nothing less than the shape of an idea. These shapes become clearly visible using another technique that Hebb could not have imagined in 1949. We can see them in living color. A positive emission tomography (PET) scan shows the exact areas of the brain that are actively involved in any thought process.

These remarkable images are beautifully consistent with Hebb's theory of specific cell assemblies corresponding to individual perceptions and thoughts. They also validate the concept, if not the precise anatomy, illustrated in Gregor Reisch's encyclopedia, *Margarita Philosophica,* published in 1504.

"Sensation" and "fantasy and imagination" do not arise from the same ventricle, as his drawing suggested, but they *do* share a common working space: shared neural ensembles in the substance of the brain. The same assemblies of neurons that are activated when you look at a hot fudge sundae are active again when you close your eyes and imagine it.

A PET scan can show you a picture of your thought processes but, with much less bother and expense, you may get an intuitive sense of these cell assemblies in operation when you are presented with the ambiguous information in Figures 10.1 and 10.2.

In response to the two-dimensional arrangement of lines in Figure 10.1, your brain constructs a three-dimensional cube. As you look at it, you can imagine either of two possible orientations: The cube may be facing down and right, or up and left. These two perceptions may alternate from one moment to the next. First one square and then another becomes the front surface of the cube as the brain "changes its mind." When one image supplants the other, the experience fits intuitively with the concept of two networks of neurons, each competing to make its own sense of the ambiguous sensory data. Because

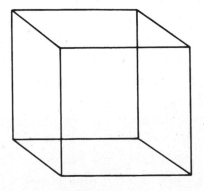

Figure 10.1

each of these cell assemblies fires as a unit, the entire image takes part in this transformation at once.

If you see a triangle in Figure 10.2, it exists only in your brain. Your ganglion cells are signaling only about the borders of three black, pie-shaped areas, each one missing a segment. Assemblies of neurons that have created three-cornered images in the past create the illusion of a triangle by filling in the frame where no contrast is reported from your eyes. The missing segments of the circles appear lighter than the rest of the page because of their stark contrast with the dark surfaces adjacent to them, and the brain paints the rest of the triangle with that same, exaggerated degree of whiteness. An assembly of neurons in your brain constructs a triangle that seems to hover above and partially cover three black circles and appears whiter than the surrounding page; a completely subjective image that combines objective clues from your eyes with your *expectation* of a triangle.

Daniel Dennett declared that "vision requires expectations,"[3] and we now know where to look for them. Expectations are built from memories, and the vaults of your memory bank lie in your associative cortex, vast expanses of cortical columns

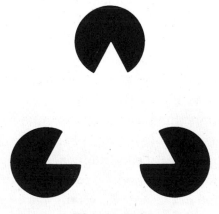

Figure 10.2

173

that are not dedicated to a specific function such as speech or vision. The safe deposit boxes that hold your individual memories are groups of neurons in your cerebral cortex, cell assemblies that were previously linked in the cooperative creation of a specific pattern of electric activity. When a portion of such an associated group of neurons is stimulated by current signals, the rest of the group will fire with them. A rough analogy would be a set of Christmas tree lights connected so that when one is lit, all will light. A current perception with some feature similar to an old one can be the switch that turns on that memory and adds its meaning to the perception at hand. When you look at a bird, a tree, or a criminal fleeing the scene of a crime, the image that you see is not simply a passive response to the light reflected to your eye. Neurons in your visual cortex synapse with networks of neurons in your associative cortex that have created similar images in the past. Those networks will fill in the missing details and create a robin, an elm tree, or a prime suspect for the district attorney based on current visual clues and past experience. Seeing a flash of blue among the leaves will activate only a diffuse assembly of neurons that have seen blue jays, balloons, and kites in a similar setting. If your retina signals the presence of enough essential details, the network of activated neurons will be more precise and may produce the image of a distinct bluebird, with all of its attendant associations and memories. This same assembly of neurons can be activated at a later time, either to re-create that memory or to embellish a dream.

Although some things are forgotten, almost everything that is not trivial does get filed away, and your brain must hold an ever-expanding collection of memories. Amazingly, there is always room for another one! This is possible because each memory is stored not as an individual, space-occupying file, but as a very specific pattern of electrical activity playing across a particular group of neurons. Just as a single violinist can play in a Shubert trio one day and in a Beethoven symphony the next, one neuron can play a part in many separate patterns. But, if space is not a problem, one would think that the retrieval of a particular memory would certainly produce a headache. Your boundless library of memories must have an impressive card catalogue, and the key to the brain's filing system is almost certainly the special neurons in the hippocampus that we considered in Chapter 6. It has long been assumed that these cells tag significant memories with distinctive, electrical call numbers, using their "memory receptors" and their unique molecular activity called long-term potentiation (LTP). Within the past three years, a dramatic wedding of genetic engineering and electrophysiological technology has made it possible to confirm that this is exactly what they do.

The gene responsible for building the "memory receptor" of the hippocampal neuron was identified and selectively eliminated from a strain of mice. All of the offspring of these mice are unable to remember where their food is hidden and fail to learn new tricks as quickly as their normal counterparts. In a second and even more dramatic experiment described in Chapter 6, an extra copy of the gene for building the memory receptor was given to another strain of mice, which the media has since dubbed smart mice because of their markedly enhanced memory and learning ability. Electrodes were placed on the specific cells in the hippocampus suspected as being responsible for that improvement, and the distinctive electrical activity of that small group of cells was observed to correlate directly with their memory-dependent behavior.[4]

Mice will not remember where their food was hidden nor learn new tricks when they are missing the gene that manufactures the "memory receptor" molecule in the hippocampus, and they will remember better and learn more easily when

175

they are given an extra copy of that gene. These experiments not only confirm that specific receptor's role in cataloguing memories for storage; they cross an important threshold that should give us pause. When it is possible through genetic manipulation to improve memory and intelligence, how will this capability be used and who will have the ability and motivation to use it? The gap between the haves and the have-nots may be soon defined in more than just material and economic terms. Hebb merely suggested that we might look for memories in the library of shifting electrical patterns in the associative cortex. Now, we are learning to enhance their production and to preordain selected mental abilities. We have reached a critical turning point with no clear view of the road ahead.

An ensemble of neurons can often be reactivated at will, as when you easily recall a scene from a movie you saw last week. But memories are recalled with varying degrees of difficulty. If you have ever run into an old acquaintance unexpectedly, someone you had not seen or thought about for several years, you may have suffered through several awkward moments exchanging pleasantries while waiting for the memory of their name to surface. Finally, something about their eyes or the tilt of their head when they laughed may have triggered that name-producing set of neurons to fire. You will recall that this happened in an instant. The entire ensemble fired at once and probably just in time to spare you an embarrassing admission. The retrieval process is not perfect. Reactivation may become difficult because of repression, confusion, or simply the passage of time. Cell assemblies can sometimes fire in odd combinations, accounting for the bizarre constructions of your dreams and the varied responses to a Rorschach test. They can be activated under hypnosis and, with appropriate suggestion, they can resurrect an actual memory or create a false one, mixing real and imagined events.

It is a difficult conceptual leap to equate an electric buzz with things as subjective as perceptions, thoughts, and memories. This leap may be easier to make if you remind yourself that less complex sets of electric signals pass through your radio, television, or CD player and regularly produce your favorite programs. In the proper machine, dots, dashes, squiggles, and bytes regularly produce messages, sounds, and sights. Perhaps the broad strip of lightbulbs that scroll news bulletins across Times Square is a better analogy than a simple string of Christmas tree lights to convey the concept of information being transmitted by the cooperation of individual neurons. The laser track etched on a computer disk is harder to see, but it comes even closer to depicting the wealth and complexity of the signals of a cell assembly. And yet, a neuron is not nearly as simple as a bulb blinking on and off or the zeros and ones that make up computer codes. Each neuron has an internal world of molecules. Each molecule follows the instructions written by accidents of mutation that proved adaptive over the millennia, as well as to contemporary experience, hormonal influences, and the commands of circulating, neuroactive chemicals. The complexity inherent in the range of activity of thousands of different molecules in one neuron, in a neuronal ensemble of tens of thousands, in a galaxy of 100 billion neurons staggers the imagination. Outside of the laboratory and scientific journals, analogies are still the best way to deal with this complexity.

It is not just the song of the neuron that matters, but which neurons sing together, and when. Neurons form associations and, like people, they are influenced by the company they keep. You behave one way on the job, another at a Saturday morning softball game, and quite another at a dinner party that evening. Similarly, the behavior of a neuron—and its effect on you—depends on the particular group of cells with which it fires. Some neural cliques, such as those for sucking and grasping, are formed at birth.

No matter which part of the newborn's palm is touched, the neuronal ensemble that is stimulated will cause all five fingers to flex. Regardless of what is brushing lightly against a newborn's cheek, its lips will pucker and begin the coordinated activity on which its survival now suddenly depends. Crawling, walking, and talking involve more complex neuronal associations that will take longer to develop. Your fingers fly across a keyboard typing letters whose relative positions were learned one by one, long ago. Repetition gradually strengthened synapses between one set of neurons that recognizes symbols and another that deftly moves your digits and still another that directs your lips, tongue, and larynx.

Strengthening synapses within a group of neurons produces a more coordinated behavior, a more developed skill and, for better or for worse, a more ingrained habit. Psychotherapy can be viewed as the difficult task of changing group allegiances. It is an attempt to weaken the synaptic bonds linking a dysfunctional, counterproductive group of neurons and strengthen synapses in those cell assemblies that produce behavior more suited to a successful adaptation to the environment. We have come a long way since mental disease was dismissed as an unexplainable, god-given curse. It can now be viewed as a manifestation of abnormal electrochemical activity, usually involving connections between the emotional, subcortical regions of the brain and the cognitive, cerebral cortex.

In 1996, abnormal patterns of activity in exactly such a circuit were observed in patients suffering from obsessive-compulsive disorder (OCD) and were seen to decrease after a favorable response to treatment—perhaps the first demonstration of a concrete, observable alteration in brain function as a result of talking therapy.[5] OCD is a mental disorder memorably portrayed by Jack Nicholson in his Oscar-winning performance in the movie *As Good As It Gets.* It is characterized by compelling, intrusive thoughts and urges that often lead to repetitive, quirky behavior such as frequent hand washing and the diligent avoidance of cracks in the sidewalk. A number of studies have linked this disorder with abnormal activity in a neural circuit connecting the orbital frontal cortex, the anterior cyngulate gyrus, and the basal ganglia. The first two of these areas are known to evaluate sensory stimuli and signal pleasure or alarm. The basal ganglia, situated near the thalamus, is implicated in the formation of habit patterns, complex behavioral responses that are mobilized rapidly with little conscious thought or awareness. PET scans done on twelve patients with symptoms of OCD showed an abnormally high level of glucose metabolism in the neural circuits connecting these three areas before treatment, and a clear-cut reduction to normal levels after successful psychotherapy had relieved their symptoms. A number of specific neuropsychiatric disorders have each been associated with unique neural circuits in the frontal subcortical region of the brain.[6] This area includes the *amygdala* (Latin for almond-shaped), which we know to be involved with aggression, fear, and alarm, and the *hippocampus,* which is intimately involved with the formation of memories and learning. All of these areas are in close communication with the thalamo-cortical pathways recently implicated by Llinás and others in a number of behavioral disorders. Psychiatrists may someday soon acquire the luxury enjoyed by other medical specialists, of being able to easily measure the progress of their patients. Observing the patterns of activity of neural ensembles may soon become tantamount to reading a mind.

11

Pure Wizardry

Matching Your Behavior to Your Situation

SOMEONE LEADING YOU by the hand and magically walking you into a neuron might very well turn to you and say, "Pay no attention to that man behind the curtain. He's a mathematician!" Within each of your branching neurons there is a mathematical wizard with a molecular bag of tricks who can give you courage, wisdom, and compassion, and who can take you to Kansas if that is where you want to go.

Neurons perform mathematical calculations nonstop, even as you sleepily reach for your morning coffee. As you scan the table to find your mug, the position of your neck, head, and eyes tell you that it is at a point x distance away from, y degrees below, and z degrees to the right of your face. Welcome back to trigonometry. Even in your groggy, prebreakfast state, your nervous system quickly transforms this sensory data into a series of motor vectors that will allow you to grasp your cup without spilling its precious contents. With neither blackboard nor chalk, neurons instantly compute the coordinates necessary for your shoulder, elbow, wrist, and fingers to put the mug handle safely in your grasp. In this example, you will have enough time to modify your action in mid-course if necessary. When you see a wine glass tipping over the edge of a table, this computation and your movement are almost instantaneous, and entirely preplanned.

The cerebellum ("little cerebrum") is a knobby projection behind the base of the brain, and is a key participant in this planning. Although not essential for movement, your cerebellum makes your moves smooth and purposeful, it is what makes you a smooth operator. Damage to the cerebellum causes awkwardness as though the various parts of a motion have to be thought of one by one, a clumsiness marked by overshooting or undershooting the endpoint. With a damaged cerebellum, your hand might first stop short of the cup and then push through it, spilling your coffee.

Dr. Rudolpho Llinás was intrigued by the fact that the neurons of the cerebellum are arranged in that familiar pattern of parallel layers we saw in the retina and the cerebral cortex. Here was another example of the order in the midst of the brain's complexity that so enthralled Ramón y Cajal when he first glimpsed its internal architecture one hundred years ago. Like Stephen Kuffler, Rudolpho Llinás followed a circuitous route to the United States. Dr. Llinás obtained his M.D. in Bogotá, Colombia, in 1959 and his Ph.D. in neurophysiology in 1965 after studying at Harvard University with Dr. Kuffler and at the Australian Institute of Advanced Studies in Canberra. He quickly rose from associate professor of physiology at the University of Minnesota in 1967 to professor and head of the neurobiology division at the University of Iowa in 1970, and has been the chief of the department of neuroscience at New York University since 1976. In 1977, he realized that the power of the computer might help

181

to explain the significance of those parallel sheets of neurons, and his hunch was right. Some very interesting things happen between those sheets! Where one neatly arranged layer of neurons meets with the next, Dr. Llinás found the interface of perception and behavior. If you define your personality as the unique way that your personal experience is translated into your own characteristic mode of behavior, then Dr. Llinás had discovered exactly where—and how—that personality is shaped. Your mannerisms and disposition are not molded in one central area, but in neatly layered sheets of neurons distributed throughout your gray matter. Your unique, reflexive way of responding to the world is wired into layered networks, whose orderly arrangement has fascinated every-one who has ever studied the brain under a microscope.

As signals pass from one layer to the next, a magical transformation takes place. Perceptions are transformed into the unique behavior that defines an individual. This metamorphosis occurs in the gray matter of the cortex as well as within several small islands of gray matter, *nuclei* and *ganglia,* deep in the brain, such as the basal ganglia, thalamus, hippocampus, pituitary, amygdala, superior colliculi, vestibular nuclei, and others. In one network, sensory signals are transformed into signals for a motor activity, in others they are converted into signals for hormonal secretion, an immune response, a memory, an idea, or an emotion. Math is probably not your native language, and I will not burden you with formulas. However, to give you an idea of how this magic is performed, I will introduce two terms that may bring back a flood of high-school memories. Mathematicians would describe the pattern of sensory signals intruding on your gray matter as an *array* of sensory *vectors*. An *array* is a number of mathematical elements arranged in a matrix, a series usually depicted in rows and columns. A *vector* is a quantity having both magnitude and direction.

When you bite into an apple, the signals from the receptors on your tongue and in your nose tell you that this is neither a peach nor a pear, but a perfectly ripe, Granny Smith apple. You perform this taste test by comparing the relative values of an array of sensory signals. Before you can say "mmm, delicious," you have calculated their matrix, calibrated their vectors, and plotted the precise coordination of sweetness, tartness, texture, and temperature that you appreciate so well. The details of this mathematical miracle make for difficult reading. It is easier and more rewarding to follow this process as you start your day.

The outer layer of the cerebellum receives a complex array of signals from every part of your body. Signals describing your body's position and orientation arrive via the spinal cord and several areas of the brain, including the gravity sensors in your inner ear. Signals describing the sight and smell of your coffee mug, the feel of the cold, hard floor under your feet and the sound of children waking nearby, radiate down from the cerebral cortex. Signals describing your sphere of special interest, your level of attention and emotional state shuttle over from the cyngulate gyrus, amygdala, hippocampus, and other subcortical areas. All of this information is coded in an array of spiking frequencies that enters the cerebellum, passes through the thick forest of the dendrites of its neurons, through their cell bodies, and is transformed into a very different set of outgoing signals. These signals leave the cerebellum as an array of vectors that will orchestrate the motor activity necessary for your appropriate, coordinated response as you simultaneously lift your cup, step onto a warm rug, turn to greet your children with a cheerful "Good morning!"—and wait for their response.

With his co-workers Pellionisz and Perkel, Rudolpho Llinás

programmed a computer with a model of a frog's cerebellum complete with 16,820 incoming sensory axons, 1.68 million intermediate cells, 8,285 output cells, and all of the appropriate connections. They showed that the cerebellar neuron performs exactly the kind of algebra necessary to accurately transform one vector array into another.[1] As signals pass from one layer of the cerebellum to the next, each neuron in the output layer performs the complex calculations necessary to compute the *matrix array* of sensory data and transform it into a new *vector* of motor signals. Between one layer and the next, perception ends and behavior begins with mathematics.

The first time a new behavior is tried, it may be a bit off the mark. Practice makes perfect, or nearly so, because as Hebb predicted, synapses get more efficient with each repetition. As similar sensory signals pass repeatedly from one layer of a network to the next, a streamlining process occurs. Synapses central to a task fire more frequently than the rest and are strengthened, while more extraneous neurons fire less consistently, produce weaker responses, and dwindle. With each repetition, fewer neurons participate and the motor task is performed with more precision and fluidity. The ancient practitioners of tai chi were absolutely right when they described their ritualized body movements as a way of directing the flow of the chi, the vital force that animates the body, and they cleverly defined the chi broadly enough to accommodate the later discovery of neural signals.

When you took the training wheels off your bicycle, it took a while to learn how far to turn the handlebars to compensate for a lean to one side. With practice, your ride became less wobbly. Each time the cerebellum repeated the transformation of sensory input regarding balance—from your joints, eyes, inner ear, and vestibular nuclei—into neural output to your muscles, only the synapses central to that specific task were strengthened. As in tai chi, your movements became more pre-cise, more nearly instantaneous, and more automatic. Before long you were able to steer very nearly a straight line without giving it a thought.

Like all of the acrobatic, beautifully coordinated, circus performances of your troupe of muscles and nerves, standing up from your chair begins with a chorus of sensory signals. Directing your attention to the center ring, sensory signals res-onate throughout your nervous system, announcing your body position and your center of gravity. They proclaim to diverse areas of your brain, including your cerebellum, that in order to avoid a very bad fall, you will need to bring your feet backward under your chair and tip your torso forward *before* you extend your legs and body into an upright position.

Action potentials arrive at your muscles from multiple centers in the spinal cord, midbrain, forebrain, cerebellum, and cerebral cortex and, once again, just as with sensory networks, there is no clear-cut, highest center. Each motor neuron takes into account neural activity throughout the nervous system and, at every moment, modifies its output so that your move-ments are smooth and purposeful. They might even reflect admonitions heard early in your life that you keep your head erect and maintain good posture. Like all of your behavior, your stance and gait are the product of your current situation as well as past experience. Your every move expresses your individuality.

Llinás, Pellionisz, and Perkel provided a mathematical framework for understanding how parallel sheets of neurons allow you to learn to ride a bicycle, perfect your golf swing, or perhaps, play the violin. These same computations also trans-form sensory signals into appropriate emotional responses. When you see the face of a loved one in a crowd, one small island of gray matter in the cyngulate gyrus instantly transforms the glimpse of that special smile into a pattern of signals that quickens your heart. A specialized group of neurons in a portion of the amygdala has evolved to transform the threatening visual image of bared teeth and a predatory scowl into the very specific emotion of fear. A patient with a lesion in this region will remain completely unperturbed when suddenly confronted by even the most menacing visage and will show no increase in activity of the adrenal gland or other visceral signs of alarm, which would normally prepare one to fight or to flee. Because of a localized injury, the amygdala does not transform this scary sensory data and the patient does not feel threatened.

A striking feature of the human brain is the number of connections between its various parts. These far outnumber its connections with sensory receptors, muscles, and glands. Most of its axons travel from one intermediate neuron to another and, as Gerald Edelman, the well-known molecular biologist and brain theorist, put it, "Your brain is more in touch with itself than with the outside world."[2] The complexity of your brain seems to be more in the service of thought than action. A spider's brain is sufficiently complex to spin stupendous, silken webs, but it lacks the interneural web of synaptic connecitons that might allow it to think about what it is doing. With its axons almost exclusively connecting sensory neurons with motor neurons, its brain is built for relfex action. Your intricate, interlacing, interneural patterns seem to be designed for introspection. By looking at its structure one could conclude that the human brain is built to figure itself out.

A clear picture of mental activity is emerging. It begins with the movement of molecules that causes electrically charged ions to pass through the cell wall of the neuron. Small changes in voltage pass along the surface of each member of a galaxy of neurons and transmit signals across synapses. Joining a chorus of others, these signals pass through multilayered columns and sheets of neurons to create carefully crafted patterns. The simplest of these patterns produces a reflex action, such as your automatic kick shortly after your doctor taps your knee. As the complexity of the patterns increases, as the numbers of neurons involved and the sizes of the neuronal ensembles expand, so do the intricacy of your resulting perceptions, the sophistication of your behaviors, and the depth of your contemplation. Taken in total, you *are* those patterns of electrical activity, and they are *you*.

12

Your Personal Chemistry

From Molecules to Moods and from Genes to Behavior

IF YOU PICK UP A CURRENT issue of a neuroscience journal there is a good chance that the lead article will try to entice you with a description of a chemical with an impossible name and the role it plays in the neuron of a sea creature you have never seen. These arcane reports are not likely to fly off the shelves at your local newsstand, yet they will have a major impact on life in the twenty-first century. They report about more than chemical reactions. They tell of the secret life of the neuron, its diet, its likes and dislikes, how it grows, the ways it communicates, and how it courts and mates with other neurons. They are teaching us the most intimate details about ourselves.

Neuropharmacology today is a bit like the carriage industry in 1905. The world of medicine is changing completely. The human genome project is speeding toward conclusion. As I write this, a team of researchers has devised a test that will reduce from years to days the time it will take to find the exact structure of a gene's expressed protein, the molecule that evolution has instructed that gene to make.[1] The possibility of understanding, preventing and curing *most diseases* is real and it is breathtaking. Gene therapy, replacing defective genes with healthy ones, has cured babies born with severe combined immune deficiency (SCID).[2] Without this treatment, these children would have been forced to live in germ-free bubbles, or worse, would die from infectious diseases that in otherwise healthy babies would cause only minor illness. By the time you read this book, clinical trials of gene therapy, stem cell transplants, and drugs designed molecule by molecule with unprecedented specificity may already be underway to treat Parkinson's disease, Huntington's disease, and a growing list of others. That we have arrived at this exciting threshold is even more astounding when you realize how we got here. It was not a promising beginning.

Prior to 1950, neurochemistry could be summed up in two words, *acetylcholine* and *norepinephrine.* Those are the two chemicals released at the nerve endings of the *autonomic nervous system.* This network of nerves is somewhat of an accessory to your central nervous system. Its nerves run down the outside of the spinal cord in a spindly chain, not inside the cord with the better protected motor and sensory nerves going to and from your brain, and that makes these auxiliary nerves a little more accessible to chemical analysis.

The autonomic nervous system is a two-part, yin and yang consortium. The yang, or active element, is the *sympathetic system.* Its nerves release norepinepherine at their nerve endings and work to speed up those functions that help you out in an emergency. They increase your heart and respiration rates and keep you at a peak of readiness. To make things easy, you just need to remember that the sympathetic system supplies norepinephrine to your adrenal gland, and everyone remembers that the adrenal gland produces the adrenaline rush that prepares

189

you for fight or flight. The *parasympathetic system* is the more passive, yin half of the equation. It releases the transmitter acetylcholine, which kicks in after a heavy meal, slows down your heart and lungs, and gets your intestines moving. It has also been shown that acetylcholine transmits impulses from motor nerves to voluntary muscles. In summary, as far as most of the world knew, there were two chemical neurotransmitters. One works only at sympathetic nerve endings, and the other works both at parasympathetic and at voluntary motor nerve endings. A medical student in 1950 didn't have to cram very hard for a neurochemistry test.

Neuropharmacology for the first half of the century was a mixture of folk remedies and jungle lore. Drugs were used because they worked, and all attempts to figure out why were severely limited by technology. A major start in the right direction came from an unlikely source. Certain jungle-dwelling South American tribes were highly feared because of the widely heralded, lethal effects of their arrows. Even a minor scratch proved fatal, rendering its perplexed and hapless victim unable to move or to breathe. The tar in which those arrowheads were dipped contained curare, a close chemical cousin to acetyl-choline. Close, but not that close. Unlike acetylcholine, curare doesn't give parasympathetic nerve endings a second look, it passes them right by, but when it reaches a motor nerve receptor, it settles in. It parks there and then does nothing. That is the problem for its victim. Curare occupies acetylcholine's motor receptor site, but it doesn't stimulate the muscle. In the meantime, acetylcholine has to keep circling the block while time runs out for a slightly wounded but totally immobile and breathless warrior. The result is a fatal paralysis. For a while, curare was actually used medically, although in small, well-measured doses, to enhance muscle relaxation in surgery, and when setting broken bones.

Similar but less gruesome stories filtered in from Europe. Belladonna (*bella* = beautiful; *donna* = lady) caught on with Italian women and earned its name because of its cosmetically pleasing effect of dilating the pupils. Like atropine, scopolamine, and other extracts from the nightshade family of plants, belladonna acts as though it stimulates the sympathetic nerves. It increases the heart rate and respiration, causes dry mouth, dilate the pupils, and causes flushing of the skin. It also quiets down the intestines and is useful for treating diarrhea. When chemical analysis became possible, it was learned that these sympathetic effects were brought about by breaking down acetylcholine at the parasympathetic receptors. With no competing parasympathetic activity, the sympathetic nerves exerted a disproportional effect. The message was loud and clear. If one could just get an idea of what those receptors and transmitters really look like and if one could design molecules like origami figures, twisted and folded to precisely fit some of those receptors, block others and, fantasy of fantasies, to replace and repair faulty ones, the possibilities would be endless.

Dr. Rita Levi-Montalcini did more than fantasize, she experimented. Her passion for behavioral science managed to elude the Nazis as well as the Allied bombardment of her hometown of Turin, Italy. She had been forced to give up her practice of neurology and psychiatry when "non-Aryans" were excluded from the professions. But, in the small bedroom in which she hid in 1941, she set up a makeshift laboratory. There, by candlelight and with curtains drawn both day and night, she discovered a remarkable extract from the nervous system of the chick embryo. This substance stimulates the growth of developing nerves and directs their differentiation and orderly maturation. Out of one of history's darkest hours she brought the discovery of nerve growth factor (NGF), a substance that regulates the growth of cells. Dr. Levi-Montalcini continued her research in cellular neurobiology for the next thirty-five years, dividing her time between a professorship at Washington University in St. Louis and the National Neurobiology Research Center in Rome, which she directed. She received a Nobel Prize in 1986 for work that has led to a new understanding of nerve cell development, the growth of cancer cells, congenital malformations, dystrophies, and new approaches to treatment. Clinical trials of a purified form of NGF are currently underway at Stanford University, where neurologist Dr. Bruce Adornato is testing its efficacy in repairing peripheral nerve damage caused by diabetes.

However, with the exception of an occasional story like that of NGF, the sad truth is that we owe much of our sophisticated knowledge of neurochemistry to serendipity. During the 1950s and 1960s, wonderful new treatments for brain diseases were discovered quite by accident. We benefited primarily from plain, dumb luck.

In 1948, in a remote hospital in Australia where he practiced psychiatry, John Cade had the idea that the wild mood swings of his patients with manic-depressive disorder might be caused by a hormone whose cyclic variation in secretion could account for those cycles of behavior. Urine was the logical place to look for hormones and, when Cade injected rats with urine samples from his patients, those animals became noticeably less active. In the course of these experiments, Cade used lithium salts to dissolve a chemical in the urine and finally realized that it was lithium and not the urine that was making his rats slow down. Since lithium salts were widely used as a substitute for table salt by people with high blood pressure, he knew it to be reasonably safe. After taking some himself to make sure that it was, he began giving lithium carbonate to a fifty-one-year-old patient who had been hospitalized for five years in a state of chronic, manic excitement. After three weeks of twice-daily doses of lithium carbonate, the patient's mania disappeared. He left the hospital, which otherwise would have been his home for life, returned to his old job, and remained well as long as he continued to take his medicine.[3] The results are not always so dramatic, but lithium remains a highly successful treatment for manic depressive disorder today—and we still don't really know how it works.

A second bit of serendipity in the 1950s truly revolutionized the practice of psychiatry and the prevailing attitudes about mental disease. The French pharmaceutical company Rhône Poulenc Laboratories was trying to synthesize a new compound to relieve symptoms of the common cold and produced chlorpromazine. This is an injectable drug very similar in structure to antihistamines, which were known to reduce coughing and sneezing. Since chlorpromazine could be given by injection prior to surgery, the neurosurgeon Henri Laborit was eager to try it on his patients. He hoped that it might prevent postoperative respiratory complications by drying secretions while at the same time facilitating general anesthesia with the mild sedative effect one would expect from an antihistamine. Anesthesiologists were delighted with its remarkable tranquilizing effect, and in 1952 two French psychiatrists, Jean Delay and Pierre Deniker, following Laborit's suggestion, administered chlorpromazine to some of their more agitated psychotic patients who were resistant to all existing therapies. After treating only ten patients, Deniker reported that he, his medical staff, and nursing personnel were stunned by the sudden transformation that had occurred. Patients previously confined to locked wards, rocking back and forth in apparent stupor, ranting at imagined voices, or lapsing into violent rage were suddenly freed of their demons.

The new drug was given the trade name Thorazine and it revolutionized the care of psychotic patients, relieving the endless torment that had often been their hopeless fate. Without any notion of how it works, psychiatrists witnessed a miracle. Previously unmanageable patients were released from locked hospital wards to return to their homes and families and were treated as outpatients. The miracle of Thorazine came at the cost of a very common side effect, but this drawback turned out to be an important clue to its mode of action. Large doses of Thorazine caused muscle rigidity very similar to that seen in patients with Parkinson's disease.

The significance of that side effect became clear when, at about the same time, three chemicals were isolated from brain tissue. Two of these, *dopamine* and *serotonin,* were new discoveries. The third, *norepinephrine,* already well known in the autonomic nervous system, was now discovered to play an important role in the brain as well. All three are fairly simple chemical compounds. Each contains a single amine group, hence their classification as *monoamines* and, because some synapses have receptors designed especially for them, these simple chemicals dramatically alter behavior.

An avenue for understanding brain chemistry was opened when it was discovered that patients with Parkinson's disease have markedly reduced levels of dopamine in their basal ganglia, a region of the brain where this monoamine is normally concentrated. This discovery eventually led to the first rational, chemical treatment of a neurological disorder, the development of a close relative of dopamine, the drug L-dopa. By replenishing the brain's supply of that depleted neuromodulator, this drug diminishes the disabling tremors and rigidity of Parkinson's disease.

This rational approach to brain chemistry was furthered by a second lucky accident in 1954. Someone at a Swiss pharmaceutical company, Ciba, got wind of a tale of Indian folk medicine. Extracts from the plant *Rauwolfia serpentina* had been used in ancient Hindu medicine to treat insomnia and insanity, and Indian physicians had noticed that it was also effective in lowering blood pressure. This is what interested Ciba. They were successful in isolating the plant's active ingredient, reserpine, and marketed it as an effective treatment for hypertension. That might have been the end of the story, except that the American psychiatrist Nathan Kline recalled the ancient Hindu reports of the tranquilizing effect of the Rauwolfia plant. Reserpine was now an approved drug, so he carefully administered it to some of his schizophrenic patients and reported their progress as they became calmer, less suspicious, and more cooperative. It was soon demonstrated that reserpine causes a marked reduction in all three monoamines: dopamine, norepinephrine, and serotonin. Because of its effect on dopamine, it shares Thorazine's side effect, a rigidity similar to that seen in Parkinson's disease.

A Swedish pharmacologist, Arvid Carlsson, took the next step. He administered Thorazine to one group of rats and reserpine to another in an attempt to establish a solid, rational link between chemistry and behavior. Thorazine and reserpine both reduce the effect of dopamine, but each in a different way. Thorazine binds to dopamine receptors, blocking dopamine's influence. Reserpine depletes dopamine from the brain. Not only were there now two effective drugs for the treatment of schizophrenia, but, for the first time, there was an understanding of how they work and a rational basis for further drug development.

In the mid-1950s, two more drugs came on the market for reasons completely unrelated to their ultimate role. They would later completely transform the treatment of severe depression. Iproniazid was developed as an antituberculosis drug and was observed to alleviate the depression of some of the patients who took it. The second, imipramine, was synthesized for purely corporate reasons, to compete with the blockbuster drug Thorazine. Because of its similar chemical structure, it was expected to behave similarly and cut into Thorazine's monopoly. Although the slight difference was enough to avoid a claim of patent infringement, it also made the new drug ineffective in the treatment of schizophrenia. However, this difference also produced the completely unexpected effect of relieving depression. Imipramine was the first of a series of drugs known as tricyclic antidepressants, which are still commonly prescribed. The mechanism of action of iproniazid and imipramine were determined only after they had been widely used for several years, and once again, monoamines were implicated in the regulation of mood.

The connection was discovered by American biochemist Julius Axelrod, who was awarded a Nobel Prize in 1970 for his pioneering work in this field. Whereas Thorazine and reserpine *decrease* monoamine activity and relieve the symptoms of *schizophrenia,* imipramine and iproniazid *increase* monoamine activity and relieve *depression.* Axelrod put science ahead of serendipity in the search for neuroactive drugs and was able to demonstrate the four possible fates of the monoamines after they are released at the synaptic membrane. The first is that they are successful in reaching and stimulating a receptor site at the opposite membrane and to transmit their signal. But there are three ways they can fail. Enzymes can degrade them; other chemicals can block them from reaching their receptors; or they can be transported back from where they came, to try another time. The last of these, reuptake, was an unexpected finding that has proved to be a boon to the drug industry and to patients. Drug companies have scrambled to capitalize on his finding that there are specific proteins continually transporting each of these monoamines back into the cells that released them. His discovery led to the production of selective

196

serotonin reuptake inhibitors (SSRIs) such as Prozac, Zoloft, and Paxil, which have far greater therapeutic effects and fewer, although different, side effects than earlier drugs.

When he made this discovery, Axelrod had been a respected but undistinguished chemist in various laboratories for twenty years, working in bacteriology, industrial hygiene, and chemical pharmacology. At the age of forty-three, he had just completed his Ph.D. and was appointed as chief of the section on pharmacology at the National Institutes of Mental Health. He had found his niche. For the next twenty-five years, Julius Axelrod played a major role in transforming psychiatry into a biologically based science, linking behavior to chemistry in a meaningful way. Detailed knowledge of the chemistry of the synapse now allows for the manufacture of custom-built compounds such as beta-blockers, alpha agonists, calcium channel blockers, and others that selectively influence receptors at particular nerve endings throughout the body. These "designer drugs" successfully treat high blood pressure, abnormal heart rhythm, glaucoma, urinary retention, and impotence by their action on autonomic nerve endings in (respectively) blood vessels, the heart, the eye, the bladder, and the penis.

There was a long and disappointing lull in the progress of neuropharmacology after the introduction of its wonder drugs a few decades ago. The blame for this can be placed squarely on two major problems, both of which seemed intractable until very recently. One is the *blood-brain barrier.* As described in Chapter 1, the membranes surrounding the brain are extremel protective of their precious contents. Molecules must be eith very small, or else shaped very precisely, to fit through filter, which, because of its effectiveness, is referred to as rier. Giving dopamine to Parkinson's patients is useless the drug circulates through the blood vessels witho into the brain tissue where it is needed. L-dopa ruse. Only a small amount of the dose that is given actually makes it into the brain, and it does not act like dopamine when it gets there. It merely stimulates the production of the real thing.

The molecules of a few drugs, such as Prozac and Thorazine, are able to cross the blood-brain barrier, but their effectiveness is limited by a second problem, the wide variety of the brain's chemical receptors and their uneven distribution. We now know that Axelrod gave us only a glimpse of a gargantuan problem. There are far more neurotransmitters and receptor types than anyone then imagined. We know of at least five separate receptors for dopamine alone, each one having a different distribution in the brain and each having different chemical affinities. Just as wine-producing grapes are grown only in certain regions, specific areas of the brain produce particular receptor proteins. As neurotransmitters circulate through the brain, they act only on those neurons with specific receptors for them. The same fine wine that sends a connoisseur into rapture may have no special impact on a beer drinker with an insensitive palate. Without the proper receptor, a neuron will similarly ignore the most potent neurotransmitter.

Giving drugs to animals was fine for observing behavioral effects but gave no clue as to which receptors were involved. One cannot easily visit the vineyards that produce neurotransmitters, which now number in the dozens, or pluck receptors like grapes. In the 1970s, Solomon Snyder at Johns Hopkins took another approach. Using radioactively labeled compounds and bits of chopped-up brain tissue from a region of interest, ne was able to identify which chemicals bind to the receptors that area. These *direct binding assays* provided information out which drugs might be effective in the brain—if the recep-ou were dealing with was a common variety. However, the em seemed hopeless as it soon became clear that there

198

were many "boutique" wineries, small groups of cells whose important but less common chemical receptors were invisible to the direct binding method. Enter genetic engineering.

The world changed dramatically in the early 1980s. The fantasies of previous decades were realized. Suddenly it was possible to study the shapes of receptor proteins in detail. By cloning them, one could make as many copies of a specific receptor as one needed in order to determine their precise architecture. Even the most hard-to-find receptors could now be analyzed, not only for their transmitter preferences, but for the exact sequence of their amino acid chain and a three-dimensional view of their origamilike structure. Neuroscience journals began to be filled with articles describing the affinity of various receptor sites for particular chemicals, not unlike a wine taster's review. Clinical journals, on the other hand, described only the practical benefits of those studies. Those two kinds of journals could just as well have been written in different languages. Basic researchers talked about direct binding assays and cloning of receptors. Not many clinicians knew or cared very much about either. However, they and their patients were very happy to reap the rewards. Behavioral psychologists also sat up and took notice.

Soon after Timothy Leary popularized the awareness that chemistry colors our view of the world as well as our behavior, neurochemistry had already become a major area of serious research. Almost as soon as it became possible to test for neurotransmitters, clinical studies began to correlate levels of serotonin and norepinephrine with repeated criminal violence and suicide. Both violent criminals and suicidal patients were found to have low serotonin levels.[4] Although norepinephrine levels were high in violent criminals, they were low in suicidal patients.[5] Low levels of serotonin and norepinephrine are each associated with potentially dangerous negative feelings. Low serotonin levels predispose to moodiness, depression, violence, and suicide. High levels of norepinephrine are associated with excitability and violence and make it more likely that anger will be expressed outward at others rather than inward. These findings bolstered the Freudian view that depression and anger are two sides of the same coin. Depression and suicide are simply anger and violence turned toward the self. The regulation of norepinephrine and serotonin is central to this quagmire of human suffering.

In October 1993, Hans G. Brunner of the Netherlands studied families with a defect in the gene responsible for making an enzyme that normally destroys excess norepinephrine. The defect is carried on the X chromosome so that only males are affected and, as expected, they have higher than normal levels of norepinephrine. All of the men with this genetic defect were prone to violent outbursts. Some had been convicted of attempted murder, arson, and rape—crimes that were noteworthy for their apparent randomness and the absence of provocation.[6] Brunner's study was a sad confirmation of similar studies of laboratory mice with a similar genetic defect, also associated with aggressive behavior and abnormally high levels of norepinephrine.[7]

In a study of children and adolescents with disruptive behavior disorders at the University of Illinois Institute for Juvenile Research, a low serotonin level was the single most accurate predictor of which youngsters would go on to commit more violent crimes or suicide.[8]

The pleasant, peaceful feelings you experience after a large meal are produced by an enzyme that converts tryptophan in your food, particularly meat and grains, into the monoamine serotonin. The director of the National Institute on Alcohol Abuse, Markku Linnoila, discovered that the gene directing production of this enzyme is defective in about 40 percent of the population. This very common genetic defect is consistent with a normal, successful life; however, when those with this defective gene are under the influence of stress or alcohol, they exhibit low serotonin levels and tend toward verbal acting out and hostility.[9] Linnoila tested 100 people who had attempted suicide more than once, and a much larger group of violent alcoholics. All of the first group and almost all of the second had the defective serotonin gene.

Every one of 1,043 prisoners convicted of arson who was studied by Dr. Linnoila had a low serotonin level, and of 58 prisoners convicted of manslaughter, low serotonin levels predicted with 84 percent accuracy those who killed again after their release. Half of the homicides committed in the United States are committed under the influence of alcohol, and this does not include the additional toll from drunk driving. Curing the chemical contributions to this epidemic is a worthy goal, and it appears to be within reach. However, there is an Orwellian aspect to this vision of the future.

If we are able to identify the causes and cures of alcohol and drug addiction, antisocial behavior, learning disorders, hyperactivity, and annoying eccentricity, at what point will the interest of the individual prevail over the competing interest of society? If we find an easily curable, chemical basis for sociopathic behavior, will we compel treatment? If chemical profiling is developed to identify those susceptible to troubled lives, will this information also be used by schools, employers, and insurance companies to limit people's opportunities? Will the chemical profiles of elected officials and candidates be made public? These questions will remain rhetorical only for a short time, and they will demand clear answers. The lull in neuropharmacological progress is over. We are on the verge of discoveries which, like gunpowder and nuclear energy, hold benefits, risks, and profound ethical dilemmas. Very soon, the social implications of these advances will vigorously compete for a place on a crowded public agenda. More than ever, science is a public concern.

Genetic engineering has put us on a fast track. Rather than tediously isolating single receptor types for testing, it is possible to clone an unlimited supply. Rather than taking wild guesses about which chemicals might affect a receptor, a gene, or a behavior, it is possible to create drugs by design. All of this is possible largely because of two discoveries whose names seem designed to permanently obscure their profound impact. Perhaps it will help if you pronounce them loudly: *restriction enzymes* and the *polymerase chain reaction* (PCR).

In 1953, when Francis Crick and James Watson determined the structure of the DNA molecule, the world was stunned into silence, marveling at this inherited, double helix of nucleotides in each of your cells that spells out all of the instructions for building your proteins and your personality. But marveling was about all that happened. Nothing very exciting or practical came from that momentous discovery until the 1970s, when restriction enzymes were discovered. Even when it is explained, that important event doesn't sound terribly exciting. Restrictive enzymes protect bacteria from viral attack by severing the string of DNA in the invading virus. The important discovery was that each restrictive enzyme searches for a particular set of letters in that string and will snip at them anywhere they find them. This revelation had three far-reaching consequences.

First, it gave birth to recombinant DNA technology, the technique at the heart of biotechnology. In 1978, in his laboratory at the University of California, San Francisco, Herbert Boyer, or rather, his *restriction enzymes,* snipped out a piece of the DNA of a bacterium, which he then replaced with a synthetic version of the human insulin gene. What happened next is history. In October 1982, a bacterium became a factory producing human insulin for Boyer's fledgling company, Genentech. This was biotechnology's first product, and it came at a time when there was growing concern about the limited supply and safety of the animal insulin then being used to treat diabetes. Restriction enzymes and recombinant DNA technology are now producing a limitless supply of human insulin and they have ended those concerns forever.

Second, restriction enzymes made it possible to create libraries of cloned brain tissue, an unlimited supply of material for studying the molecular structure of even the most hard-to-find, "boutique" neuroreceptors. Neurochemistry and the search for new drugs were transformed from esoteric pursuits into practical technologies.

Third, with restriction enzymes it is possible to locate and identify specific genes within the chromosome, and the human genome project became a possibility rather than a distant dream. Your long string of genetic material could now be reduced to bite-sized chunks and studied efficiently. In 1980, in a bold paper with the not-so-bold title *Construction of a Genetic Linkage Map in Man Using Restriction Fragment Length Polymorphism,*[10] David Botstein and his co-workers began the human genome project to determine the precise spelling of your 3 billions of bits of genetic code.

The idea of the *polymerase chain reaction* (PCR) came to Kary Mullins during a drive in the California mountains in 1985. It was an idea that won a Nobel Prize in 1993. Polymerase is the enzyme that makes a second copy of a chromosome before any of your cells divide, ensuring that each of the two daughter cells has a full complement of genes. Polymerase copies every letter in the DNA chain verbatim. Kary Mullins devised a way for polymerase to do the same thing in a test tube, even with only a tiny fragment of DNA, and do it repeatedly in a chain reaction. After two repetitions there would be four copies of the DNA fragment, after three repetitions, eight strands of DNA, after twenty repetitions, more than a million, and after thirty repetitions, which can be done in less than three hours, more than a billion exact copies of the original strand of DNA are produced! PCR is what makes it possible to identify a criminal suspect from a single piece of hair and to re-create the genetic material of long-extinct animals, the premise of the movie *Jurassic Park*. This technique accelerated the pace of genetic research and the human genome project exponentially.

That was good news for Nancy Wexler. Her mother had Huntington's disease, a brain disease that affects one out of every twenty thousand people. It is an awful, untreatable disease, producing progressive dementia, depression, uncontrolled choreoform movements, and death. Its symptoms do not usually appear until well into adulthood—and it is inherited. Nancy and her sister Alice each had a fifty-fifty chance of getting that fatal, dominant gene from their mother. In 1982, Nancy Wexler and a team of researchers traveled to a remote village in Venezuela where hundreds of people were afflicted with the disease that they had inherited from a single, common ancestor. The expedition was funded by the Hereditary Disease Foundation, which included her father Milton Wexler, Jennifer Jones Simon and Norton Simon, and Marjorie Guthrie, whose folksinger husband, Woody, had died of Huntington's disease and whose son Arlo was at risk. The purpose was to collect blood samples from as many affected villagers as possible in order to study their DNA.

They would need to test a large number of people known to have the disease if their findings were to be significant, and without a complete map of the human genome, they would need to be very lucky to find the gene that was the culprit. They were. Using restrictive enzymes and its even faster offshoot, a technique called restrictive fragment length polymorphisms (RFLPs), they found the gene for Huntington's disease sitting on the upper tip of chromosome number four. That as yet incurable disease is caused by an expanded region of repeating letters g (glutamine) on a segment of DNA. Because of this glitch in their DNA's alphabetic instructions, these unfortunate souls produce a faulty protein, huntington. It is reasonable to expect that finding that defective protein and learning about its insidious activity in the brain will lead to a cure.

In November 1999, the prospects of doing just that improved remarkably. Researchers at the University of Rochester announced a new technique for finding the protein molecule produced or, in the language of biologists, expressed by a particular gene. The new technique, which involves chemically tagging individual genes and looking for the chemical tags in the expressed protein, reduces one of the most arduous tasks in biomedical research to a series of simple steps that can be completed in a few days. The implications are startling. It soon will be not only possible, but much easier than previously thought, to identify the protein molecule expressed by any gene of interest. With that information, pharmaceutical companies will be able to design drugs with a molecular structure tailored to a specific target. In addition to quickly identifying genes and the molecules they express, this technique will enable us to easily screen for drugs, addictive chemicals, pollutants in the air, water, and workplace, and to learn their effects on living cells.[11] We will no longer have to wait for lucky accidents. We will have the tools to identify the faulty protein responsible for each biological mistake, and to correct it.

In a few decades, we have gone from wild guesses and folklore to a systematic study of the chemical components of the brain's ion channels, chemical messengers, transmitters, and receptors. In the process, we have been lucky enough to produce

205

some drugs that ameliorate psychoses, depression, manic-depressive (bipolar) disease, Parkinson's disease, and myasthenia gravis. With molecular engineering and recombinant DNA technology we will now be aiming at these tiny targets with a marksman's rifle rather than a shotgun. Genetic engineering has already modified a receptor in a tiny area of a mouse's brain and enhanced both memory and learning ability.[12] It is possible to genetically alter fetal cells and even a patient's own skin and muscle cells to deliver neuroactive molecules directly into the brain or spinal cord where they are needed, bypassing the blood-brain barrier and eliminating the risk of rejection.

The cells that line the brain's ventricles, the stem cells that we now know provide a fresh, daily supply of neurons to the cortex, are even more surprising. They not only develop into cortical neurons; they will mature into whatever cell type surrounds them. Stem cells have been harvested from aborted embryos and, when placed individually into diseased heart, muscle, or nerve tissue, will not only mature into healthy, normally functioning heart, muscle or nerve cells but will also organize themselves to fit and function normally in the organs where they are placed. Christopher Reeve, the actor whose traumatic quadriplegia is a promising target of stem cell research, recently testified before a committee of the U.S. Congress, pleading that this work not be banned by those who see it through the narrow lens of abortion rights politics.

These stunning, recent advances are to neuropharmacology what the telegraph key was to telecommunication. They only hint at the potential. Along with their obvious medical benefits, they will challenge us to make judicious use of our newfound abilities to test for and to treat antisocial traits, to enhance intelligence, and to micromanage behavior. If we can wisely balance the often competing interests of society and the individual, we will have truly earned our self-congratulatory name, Homo sapiens.

13

The Final Chord

THE ASTONISHING NEWS is that—after centuries of wild speculation as to what and where it might be—we are getting our first glimpse of the mind. We have traveled through a forest that holds it tentatively in its branches. Charged bits of stardust chattering through a lush overgrowth of synapses define your world, your personality, and your personal version of humanity. Within the dark confines of your skull, the orchestrated signals of 100 billion neurons create a rich rendition of your surroundings and, in an untidy thicket of neural pathways, they lend exquisite form to your behavior. The faint music of a galaxy of neurons transforms your chaotic collisions with clouds of electrons and deflected photons into meaningful perceptions and orderly thoughts. And we have found nothing supernatural here. Awe-inspiring and worthy of wonder, certainly, but natural nevertheless. Like ions everywhere, those bits of stardust that move across your neural membranes and make you tick, their charges, electrons, and quarks all agreeably conform to nature's laws.

Your mind is not a supernatural visitor breathing life into natural flesh, as envisioned by Galen and Descartes. It is a natural and inseparable property of your brain and body. It can be plainly seen in a joyful, completely involuntary, upward pull of your facial muscles, a spring in your step, a backward tilt of your neck, the flushing of your skin, and the racing of your heart. In an instant, your mind can change to produce a flaccid face, a sagging of your shoulders and a pallor of your skin. It can lower your metabolism, diminish the flow of your hormones, reduce your immune response, cause illness, and even death. Joy can make you soar, and grief *can* break your heart.[1]

But to say that there is no separation between the mind and the body does not end the mystery. Our current understanding of how the brain works has not begun to explain the enigmatic products of the brain *as we experience them.* The neurosurgeon Dr. Peter G. Petty likens our state of knowledge to that of a television technician observing the electrical activity inside the set: "While the activity can be very precisely described, it would be impossible to tell from the waveforms whether the information received was the evening news or *The Simpsons.*"[2]

We need to step back and get a new perspective. Seeing and being are vastly different from anything we have yet found "inside the set." The objective events that flow from the infinitesimal force of a single photon and the oscillations of thalamic nuclei may correlate with our subjective experiences, but they tell us little about them. We give names such as *qualia* and *epiphenomena* to the experiential products of our brains just as physicists a century ago invented the *ether* to accommodate their ignorance of the way light travels. Like a flame leaping from embers, a powerful sense of self springs from minute molecules. This dynamic emergence strives constantly for expression and it remains for us, as it was for our cave-painting ancestors, the driving force behind our art and our passion. A single personality emanates from the enigmatic songs of countless neurons—and this powerful process remains unexplained. The goal of neuroscience is to understand the wondrous, final chord that blends the internal and external world into your singular experience of being alive.

As the twentieth century began, studying the baffling behavior of light changed our view of time and space and revealed the strange, quantum nature of the atom. Our contemporary puzzle is the perplexing emergence of order from complexity. Beyond the study of light, beyond quanta and quarks, lies the science of complex, adaptive systems. Complex mental properties emerge from the actions of single neurons and the movements of the molecules within them. A culture, with its distinctive economic, political, and social fabric, emerges from a group of individuals acting independently. Galaxies emerge from cosmic dust. Purpose and beauty emerge from invisible particles like rainbows playing in the spray of a waterfall. In every complex adaptive system, its individual components have the paradoxical ability to be independent— and yet massively interdependent—simultaneously, just as a single packet of light behaves both as a wave and a particle at the same time. We are still reeling from the unexpected consequences of trying to solve the riddle of the photon's behavior. It is impossible to guess the revelations that will flow from the solution to our current puzzle.

Our grandparents were thrilled when the carefully timed dots and dashes of a telegraph key sent personal messages to a distant city. By adding a degree of complexity, their grandchildren tap ones and zeros through a Pentium chip and send satellites to sample Saturn's rings. Kuffler recorded the carefully timed impulses of the neuron. Dowling, Hubel, and Wiesel gave us our first glimpse of the complex patterns that those signals create as they traverse your neural networks. Llinás and others are showing us how behavior, usually deft and purposeful, sometimes bizarre and unbidden, flows from a turbulent, back-propagating, stream of neuronal communication. And somehow, out of this incomparable complexity, comes consciousness.

Complex adaptive systems are now the subject of intense study in a variety of scientific venues such as the Santa Fe Institute,[3] founded by Dr. Murray Gell-Mann, who is best known for his Nobel Prize–winning discovery of the subatomic entities that he named quarks.[4] Experts in widely diverse fields are beginning to study the mystifying emergence of meaningful patterns from the freewheeling yet interdependent components of our cosmos, our societies, and our selves. Science is beginning to ask questions about chaos and order previously posed only by philosophers and religious scholars.

This is truly a remarkable time to be alive. After a few millennia of speculating on the nature of life and the universe, we have finally begun to develop proper investigative tools. We have learned more about our place in the universe and discovered more about ourselves in the last few years than in all the time that has gone before. Although we have made the humbling discovery that we are made of the same stuff as everything around us, neuroscience is applying the rigor of the laboratory to discover what makes us unquestionably unique. Are your consciousness, ecstasy, and pain the result of nothing more than the electrochemical music at the cell walls of your neurons? Is there no reason to believe in an eternal soul?

To fear that science detracts from the wonder of life is to misunderstand science. There is wonder enough in nature to make the supernatural superfluous. Hard, dry science tells us that we move to the ebb and flow of the ageless embers of long-dead stars whose electrons whirl endlessly within the temporary confines of our bodies. We dance to rhythms played on the membranes of cells that have been dividing in an unbroken succession since the first were formed in an ancient sea. As we gaze at a canopy of stars, there is an enduring intimacy between their twinkle and our nod.

In the final analysis, there is no compelling reason to hastily relinquish long-held and cherished beliefs. We have an incomplete accounting of the energy, particles, and, according to some, the vibrating, multidimensional strings that fill our universe. The light-speed travel of the photon is a constant reminder that we live in a universe where it is possible for distances to vanish and for time to stand still, where ephemeral separateness can and does give way to a timeless unity. Those ambassadors from distant stars have taught us that there is more around us than meets the eye.

Forty years ago John Kennedy stirred a nation with his call for "mastery of the sky and the rain, the ocean and the tides, the far side of space and the inside of men's minds." Since then, we have discovered how interrelated the components of those separate spheres truly are. It is no longer possible to tell separate stories of space and time, of matter and energy, of the mind and the body. To speak of one is to speak of them all. The key to grasping the wonder around us, and to fully understanding what makes us tick, appears to lie in the hint of order amid the complexity first glimpsed through the microscope of Santiago Ramón y Cajal a brief century ago. Whether by improbable accident or by incalculable plan, our brain seems uniquely designed to find that key.

Notes

Introduction

1. Paul Churchland, *The Engine of Reason: The Seat of the Soul.* (Cambridge, Massachusetts: MIT Press, 1996).

1 Exploring a Recently Discovered Galaxy

1. Francis Crick, *The Astonishing Hypothesis* (New York: Touchstone Books, 1994), 3.

2. J. Offroy de La Mettrie, *L'homme machine* 1748 (trans. from the French of the Marquis d'Argens and printed for W. Owen, London, 1749).

3. S. Ramón y Cajal, *The Cerebral Cortex: An Annotated Translation of the Complete Writings* (trans. and ed. by Javier DeFelipe and Edward G. Jones, New York: Oxford University, 1988).

4. H. Sontheimer, "Glial activity," *Journal of Neuroscience* 14: 2464–2475, May 1994.

5. Antonio Damasio, *Descartes' Error* (New York: G. P. Putnam's Sons, 1994.)

6. A.C. Crombie, "Early concepts of the senses and the mind," *Scientific American* (May 1994), reprinted in *Reading from Scientific American, Perception: Mechanisms and Models* (San Francisco: W. H. Freeman & Co., 1972).

7. W. Penfield, *The Cerebral Cortex of Man* (New York: Macmillan, 1950).

8. M. Gazzaniga, J. Bogen, and R. Sperry, "Observations on visual perception after disconnection of the cerebral hemispheres in man," *Brain,* 88:221–236, 1965.

213

9. F. R. Wilson, *The Hand: How Its Use Shapes the Brain, Language, and Human Culture* (New York: Pantheon Books, 1998).

2   Stardust and the Music of the Neuron

1. For a more detailed account see Gordon Shepard, *Neurobiology,* 1993.

2. S. Berretta and A. Graybiel, *Journal of Neurophysiology* 68: 776–777, September 1992.

3. E. Clarke and C. D. O'Malley, *The Human Brain and Spinal Cord: A Historical Study Illustrated by Writings from Antiquity to the Twentieth Century,* (University of California Press: Berkeley and Los Angeles, 1968), 206.

4. Brian Greene, *The Elegant Universe* (New York: W. W. Norton & Co., 1991).

5. E. S. Hodgson, "Taste receptors," *Scientific American,* May 1961, 135–144, and J. E. Amoore, "Sterochemical theory of odor," *Scientific American,* February 1964, 42–49.

6. A. G. Brown, *Nerve Cells and Nervous Systems* (London: Springer-Verlag, 1991).

7. A. Frazer, *Biological Bases of Brain Function* (New York: Raven Press, 1994).

8. R. Lauer, "EEG based control of a hand grasp neuroprosthesis," *NeuroReport* 10:1767–1771, June 1999.

9. N. Birbaumer, "A spelling device for the paralysed," *Nature* 398:297–298, March 25, 1999.

10. H. Eichenbaum and J. Davis, *Neuronal Ensembles: Strategies for Recording and Decoding* (New York: Wiley-Liss, 1998).

3   The Ghost in the Machine

1. E. Gould and C. Gross, "Neurogenesis in the neocortex of adult primates," *Science* 286:584–552, October 1999.

2. S. Quartz, from an essay in *The New Brain,* www.feedmag.com, June 1999.

3. B. Libet, "Unconscious cerebral initiative and the role of conscious will in voluntary action," *Behavioral and Brain Sciences* 8: 529–566, December 1985.

4. Francis Crick, *The Astonishing Hypothesis* (New York: Touchstone, 1994), 266.

5. Daniel C. Dennett, *Consciousness Explained* (Boston: Little Brown, 1991).

6. J. C. Eccles, "Do mental events cause neural events analogously to the probability fields of quantum mechanics? *Proc. Roy. Soc. Lond.* B 227:411–428, May 1986.

7. J. C. Eccles, *Evolution of the Brain: Creation of the Self* (Basingstoke, UK: Routledge, 1989).

8. R. Penrose, *Shadows of the Mind: A Search for the Missing Science of Consciousness* (Oxford, UK: Oxford University Press, 1996).

9. G. M. Edelman, *The Remembered Present: A Biological Theory of Consciousness* (New York: Basic Books, 1989).

10. M. Gazzaniga, *The New Brain,* www.feedmag.com, June 1999.

11. *Journal of Consciousness Studies.* See especially Volume 6, August/September 1999.

4 The Photon and Your Brain

1. David H. Hubel, *Eye, Brain, and Vision* (Scientific American Library, No. 22) (New York: W. H. Freeman & Co., 1995).

2. Daniel C. Dennett, *Consciousness Explained* (Boston: Little Brown, 1991).

3. See any standard physics text re: "time dilation" and "Lorentz contraction."

5 The Intelligence of the Neuron

1. David H. Hubel, *Eye, Brain, and Vision* (Scientific American Library, No. 22) (New York: W. H. Freeman & Co., 1995).

2. J. E. Dowling, *The Retina: An Approachable Part of the Brain* (Cambridge, Massachusetts: Belknap Press, 1987).

6   The Moving Parts of Your Brain

1. The molecular response to the photon was elucidated by teams of investigators led by Lubert Stryer and Anita Zimmerman at Stanford University, Palo Alto; Laurence Haynes and King-Wai Yau at the University of Texas, Galveston; and Evgeniy Fesenko at the Academy of Sciences, Moscow.

2. Zach W. Hall, *An Introduction to Molecular Neurobiology* (Sunderland, Massachusetts: Sinauer Associates, Inc., 1992).

3. Y. Tang, J. Tsien, et al., "Genetic enhancement of learning and memory in mice," *Nature* 401: 63–69, September 2, 1999.

4. N. Wade, "Scientist Creates a Smarter Mouse," *New York Times,* September 2, 1999, 1.

5. Zach W. Hall, op. cit.

6. Ibid.

7. A. D. Roses, K. H. Weisgraber, and Y. Christen, "Apolipoprotein and Alzheimer's Disease," *Research and Perspectives in Alzheimer's Disease* (Berlin: Springer Verlag, 1996).

8. M. Citron, "β-secretase cleavage of Alzheimer's amyloid precursor protein by the transmembrane aspartic protease BACE," *Science,* 286:735–741, October 22, 1999.

7   The Yellow Brick Road

1. David H. Hubel, *Eye, Brain, and Vision* (Scientific American Library, No. 22) (New York: W. H. Freeman & Co., 1995).

8   The Emerald City

1. Wm. H. Dobelle, Ph.D., Columbia-Presbyterian Medical Center, New York.

2. M. Patrice Some, *Of Water and the Spirit: Ritual, Magic, and Initiation in the Life of an African Shaman* (New York: Penguin, 1995).

3. N. Tinbergen, *The Herring Gull's World* (New York: Basic Books, 1960).

4. M. Cheour, "Development of language-specific phoneme rep-

resentations in the infant brain," *Nature Neuroscience* 1:351–353, September 1998.

5. A. Gopnik, *The Scientist in the Crib, Minds, Brains, and How Children Learn* (New York: William Morrow, 1999).

6. Ibid.

7. Drs. Saul Schanberg at Duke University and Tiffany Field at the University of Miami.

8. S. Blakeslee, *New York Times,* February 2, 1999, reporting on the work of Dr. Delaina Walker Batson, University of Texas, Dallas, and Dr. Dennis Feeney, University of New Mexico, Albuquerque.

9. Brian Kolb, *Brain Plasticity and Behavior* (Mahwah, New Jersey: Lawrence Erlbaum Associates, Inc., 1995).

10. I. Gottesman, *Schizophrenia Genesis* (New York: W. H. Freeman, 1991).

11. R. L. Suddath et al., "National Institute of Health study," *New England Journal of Medicine* 322:789–794, March 1990.

12. Robin Kar-Moore and Meredith S. Wiley, *Ghosts from the Nursery: Tracing the Roots of Violence* (Boston: Atlantic Monthly Press, 1998).

9 Beyond the Yellow Brick Road

1. E. H. Land, "Recent advances in retinex theory and some implications for cortical computations," *Proc. Natl. Acad. Sci. USA* 80:5163–5169, August 1983.

2. S. Zeki, *A Vision of the Brain* (Oxford, UK: Blackwell Science, Inc., 1993).

3. Donald O. Hebb, *The Organization of Behavior* (New York: Wiley, 1949).

4. Ibid.

5. R. Eckhorn et al., "Coherent oscillations," *Biol. Cybern.* 60: 121–130, February 1988.

6. W. Singer, "Stimulus-specific neuronal oscillations in orientation columns of cat visual cortex," *Proc. Natl. Acad. Sci. USA* 86:1698–1702, 1989.

7. Francis Crick, *Astonishing Hypothesis* (New York: Touchstone Books, 1994).

8. D. Chopra, *Perfect Health* (New York: Harmony Books, 1991).

NOTES9. R. Llinás, "Thalamocortical dysrhythmia: a neurological and neuropsychiatric syndrome characterized by magnetoencephalography," *Proc. Natl. Acad. Sci. USA* 96:15222–15227, December 1999.

10 The Shape of an Idea

1. Paul Churchland, *The Engine of Reason: The Seat of the Soul* (Cambridge, Massachusetts: MIT Press, 1996). An excellent overview of artificial intelligence and computer models of the brain.
2. H. Eichenbaum and J. Davis, *Neuronal Ensembles: Strategies for Recording and Decoding* (New York: Wiley-Liss, 1998).
3. Daniel C. Dennett, *Consciousness Explained* (Boston: Little Brown, 1991).
4. Y. Tang, J. Tsien, et al., "Genetic enhancement of learning and memory in mice," *Nature* 401: 63–69, September 2, 1999.
5. A. B. Schwartz, P. W. Stoessel, et al., "Cerebral changes after successful behavior modification treatment of obsessive-compulsive disorder," *Arch. Gen. Psychiatry* 53:109–113, 1996.
6. J. L. Cummings, "Frontal-subcortical circuits and human behavior," *Arch. Neurol.* 50:873–880, August 1993.

11 Pure Wizardry

1. A. Pellionisz, R. Llinás, and D. H. Perkel, "A computer model of the cerebellum of the frog," *Neuroscience* 2:19–39, January 1977.
2. G. Edelman, *Bright Air, Brilliant Fire* (New York: Basic Books, 1992).

12 Your Personal Chemistry

1. M. Martzen et al., "A biochemical genomics approach for identifying genes by the activities of their products," *Science* 286: 1153–1155, November 5, 1999.

218

2. A. Fischer and M. Cavazanna-Calvo, "Gene therapy of human severe combined immunodeficiency (SCID)-XI disease," *Science,* 288:669–672, April 28, 2000.

3. S. Barondes, *Molecules and Mental Illness* (Scientific American Library, No. 4) (New York: W. H. Freeman, 1993).

4. G. Brown and F. Goodwin, National Institutes of Health.

5. Marie Asberg, Karolinska Hospital, Stockholm.

6. H. G. Brunner, "Abnormal behavior associated with a point mutation in the structural gene for monoamine oxidase A," *Science* 262:578–580, October 22, 1993.

7. Olivier Cases, "Aggressive behavior and altered amounts of brain serotonin and norepinepherine in mice lacking MAOA," *Science* 268:1763–1766, June 23, 1995.

8. Markus J. Kruesi, Chief of Child Psychiatry, University of Illinois Institute for Juvenile Research, Chicago.

9. R. Kotulak, *Inside the Brain* (Kansas City, MO: Andrews McMeel Publishing, 1996).

10. D. Botstein et al., "Construction of a genetic linkage map in man using restriction fragment length polymorphism," *American Journal of Human Genetics* 32:314–331, 1980.

11. M. Martzen, et al., op. cit.

12. Y. Tang, J. Tsien, et al., "Genetic enhancement of learning and memory in mice," *Nature* 401: 63–69, September 2, 1999.

13   The Final Chord

1. Paraphrased from Antonio Damasio, who pieced together the skull and the history of Phineas Gage (Chapter 1), *Descartes' Error* (New York: G. P. Putnam's Sons, 1994).

2. P. G. Petty, "Consciousness: A neurosurgical perspective," *Journal of Consciousness Studies* 5:95, September/October 1998.

3. Santa Fe Institute, 1399 Hyde Park Road, Santa Fe, NM 87501 (www.santafe.edu).

4. Murray Gell-Mann, *The Quark and the Jaguar: Adventures in the Simple and the Complex* (New York: W. H. Freeman, 1994).

Index

acetylcholine, 189, 190
actin, 114–115, 116
action potentials:
   electric signals of, 49–50
   synapse and, 58
Adornato, Bruce, 192
aging, brain and, 143
agriculture, development of, 11
aldosterone, biological clock, 123
allergens, 55, 57
alpha waves, electroencephalography, 61
Alzheimer, Alois, 116
Alzheimer's disease:
   education, 143
   molecular action, 116–118
   visual flow, 152
amino acids:
   beta-secretase, 117
   molecular action, 103–109
   visual pigment, 111
amygdala, functions of, 40, 41
amyloid plaques, Alzheimer's disease, 117
anesthesia, 193
animal domestication, development of, 11
antidepressants, 196–197
apolipoprotein E3, Alzheimer's disease, 117
Aristotle, 56
array of sensory vectors, 182–183, 184
art, light and, 80
artificial intelligence, 169
artificial vision, surgery for, 132–133
atmosphere, light, 84
atropine, 191
attention, thalamus, 162–163
auditory input. *See* hearing
Australopithecine anamensis, 12
autonomic nervous system:
   chemistry of, 189
   described, 189–190
   fetal, 81
autoradiology, development of, 120–121
Axelrod, Julius, 196–197, 198
axons:
   development of, 126–127
   white matter, 20
Baars, Bernard, 66

balance:
   evolution of, 55–56
   motion and, 150
Baum, L. Frank, 5
bees, timekeeping by, 121–122
behavior:
   brain, 73
   brain lateralization, 37–38
   neuronal ensembles, 178
   perception, 182
   subjective experience, 137
Beling, Ingeborg, 121
Belladonna, 191
Berger, Hans, 61, 62
beta-secretase, molecular action, 116–117
binding problem, brain function, 160–165
binocular vision, brain, 126
biofeedback, electroencephalography, 62–63
biological clock:
   retina, 121
   space/time continuum, 123–124
   supra-chiasmatic nucleus (SCN), 122–123
   universality of, 121–122
biology, electricity and, 26
bipolar cells, vision, 89–90
Birbaumer, Niels, 63
birds, 122, 123
blindness:
   childhood, 139
   superior colliculi and, 127–128
   surgery for, 132–133
blood-brain barrier:
   cerebrospinal fluid, 22
   pharmacology, 197–198
body/mind relationship. *See* mind/body relationship
Bois-Reymond, Emil du, 26
Botstein, David, 203
Boyer, Herbert, 202, 203
brain cells, generation of, 69–70
brain function. *See also* specific brain structures
   binding problem, 160–165
   disease, 3–4 (*See also* brain injury and disease; mental disorders; specific diseases)

free will, 70–72
hormones, 57
illusion, 72–73
neuronal communications, 21–23, 30–31
neuronal electric signals, 49–50
neurons, 7–8 (*See also* neurons)
patterns, 133–136, 186–187
reaction time, 41
sensory stimulation, 139
species-specific, 53–54
subjective experience, 4, 8–10 (*See also* subjective experience)
vision and, 81, 87–88, 93–94
brain hemispheres. *See* brain lateralization
brain injury and disease:
cerebellum, 181
illusion, 72
localization, 5
memory, 111–114
personality, 28–29
speech, 29–30
thalamo-cortical signals, 164–165
vision, 30, 151–152
visual cortex, 156–157
visual neural pathways, 153–154
brain lateralization:
behavior, 37–38
body, 30
communications in brain, 34–36
consciousness, 74
evolution, 37
brain mapping:
autoradiology, 121
historical perspective on, 23–40
subjective experience, 67–69
brain research, historical perspective, 13–20
brain stem, described, 19
brain stimulation, brain mapping, 32
brain structure. *See also* specific brain structures
cerebral cortex, 131, 157
childhood, 140–141
described, 18–23
as hierarchy, 155
neuronal ensembles (cell assemblies), 169–170
retina, 81–83 (*See also* eye; retina)
brain tumor, imaging of, 15, 16
brain ventricles. *See* ventricles
Broca, Paul, 29–30
Broca's area, language development, 140
Brodmann, Korbinian, 31
Brunner, Hans G., 200
Bush, George H. W., 64

Cade, John, 192
Cajal, Santiago, 13–14, 115, 181, 211
calcium ions:
cell potentials, 43
synapse, 58, 59
calmodulin, molecular action, 113–114
Carlsson, Arvid, 195

Carroll, Lewis, 9
CAT scans, development of, 15–16
cell assemblies. *See* neuronal ensembles (cell assemblies)
cell potentials, ions, 43
central nervous system, fetal, 81
cerebellum:
motion, 181, 185
neurons, 181–182
perception, 183–187
cerebral cortex:
described, 18, 20
infancy, 138
patterns, 134
structure of, 131, 157
cerebrospinal fluid, function of, 22
Chalmers, David, 66
chemically gated ion channels:
function of, 47
molecular action, 106
chemical messenger molecule:
chemically gated ion channels, 47
molecular action, 105
neurons, 102
chemical receptors, species-specific brain function, 54–55
chemical transmitters. *See* transmitter chemicals
chemistry, sodium-potassium pump, 44
childhood:
brain development, 140–141, 144–145
nurturing and, 146–147
visual cortex, 138–139
chloride ions, cell potentials, 43
chlorpromazine, 193
Churchland, Patricia, 100
Churchland, Paul, 1, 100
circadian rhythm. *See* biological clock
cocaine, neuronal response to, 48
cognition, neuronal ensembles, 177
color, light and, 158, 159–160
color vision:
ganglion cells, 95
visual cortex injury, 156–157
complex adaptive systems, 209–210
computer:
as metaphor, 38–39, 157
neural network computer, 167–169
cones, light perception, 85–86
consciousness:
brain lateralization and, 74
studies in, 66–67, 74–75
uncertainty principle and, 74
coordination, neurons, 180–181
corpus callosum, epilepsy surgery, 34, 35
cortex. *See* cerebral cortex
cortical neurons, visual cortex and, 130–131
cortisol, biological clock, 123
Crick, Francis, 9, 73, 161–162, 164, 202
crime:
child neglect and, 146–147
pharmacology, 199–201

culture, brain development, 141
curare, 190

Damasio, Antonio, 29
Damasio, Hanna, 29
Darwin, Charles, 52, 53, 158
Davis, Joel L., 65
daylight. *See* light
decision-making process, brain, 73
Delay, Jean, 193
delta waves, electroencephalography, 61, 62
dendrite, synapse and, 58
Deniker, Pierre, 193
Dennett, Daniel C., 66, 73, 88, 173
depolarization, ion channel selectivity, 48–49
depression, 195–197
depth perception, brain, 126
Descartes, René, 5, 25–26, 68, 73, 207
determinism, free will and, 74. *See also* free will
diet, amino acids, 104
direct binding assays, 198
disease, brain function and, 3–4. *See also*
   brain injury and disease; mental disorders; specific diseases
DNA. *See also* inheritance
   genetic engineering, 202–205
   limits of, 126
   memory receptors, 175–176
   molecular action and, 102–103, 104
   molecular structure, 202
   neuron and, 48, 65
   proteomics, 118–119
   subjective experience and, 145
dominant hemisphere, 36
dopamine, 60, 194, 195, 197–198
Dowling, John, 5, 97–99, 100, 209
dreaming:
   function of, 71–72
   neuronal ensembles, 176
   rapid-eye-movement sleep, 61–62
Dualism, Descartes, 25–26

ear. *See* hearing
earth, time line of, 10
Eccles, John, 74, 91
Edelman, Gerald, 74, 186
education, Alzheimer's disease, 143
Eichenbaum, Howard, 65
Einstein, Albert, 5, 21, 22, 78–80, 123–124
electricity, biology and, 26, 43
electroencephalography:
   biofeedback, 62–63
   development of, 61
   sleep studies, 61–62
electron microscope, research advances, 14, 43
electroshock therapy, effects of, 69, 164
embryo. *See* fetal development
emergent property, subjective experience and,
   69
emotion:
   brain and, 22–23, 40
   cerebral cortex, 134

neurons, 185–186
endocrine system:
   biological clock, 122
   brain function and, 57
environment:
   evolution and, 12–13
   heredity and, 136–137
   survival and, 11–12
ependymal cells, brain cell generation, 70
epilepsy, surgery for, 34, 35
epiphenomenon, 208
ether, 51
ethics, pharmacology, 201–202
event-related potentials (ERPs), language
   development, 140
evolution:
   balance, 55–56
   brain lateralization and, 37
   color recognition, 158–159
   environment and, 12–13
   neuron, 46
   photon and, 81, 83
   species-specific brain function, 53–54
excitable cell, defined, 45
eye, 2. *See also* retina; vision
   evolution of, 56
   motion and, 149–153
   movement of, 149
   perception and, 51–52
   rapid-eye-movement sleep, 61–62
eyesight. *See* vision

face recognition, infancy, 135
fantasy, neuronal ensembles, 172
fetal development:
   axons, 126–127
   retina, 81, 82
   visual cortex, 125–126
fetal stem cells, 206
fitness, survival and, 11–12
Freeman, Walter, 66
free will:
   brain and, 70–72, 73
   determinism and, 74
Freud, Sigmund, 137, 200
Frisch, Karl von, 121
frontal lobe:
   subjective experience, 69
   visual neural pathways, 153–154
frontal lobotomy, effects of, 69
Frost, Robert, 169
functional magnetic resonance imaging
   (FMRI), development of, 16

Gage, Phineas, 28–29, 39
Galen of Pergamum, 5, 16–18, 19, 20, 22, 25,
   26, 43, 45, 68, 70, 207
Galileo, 83
Gall, Franz, 26–27, 28
Galvani, Luigi, 26
gamma-aminobutyric acid (GABA), trans-
   mitter chemicals, 100

ganglion cells:
  receptive fields of, 91–98
  vision, 89–90
gated ion channels:
  neuron, 47
  synapse and, 59
Gazzaniga, Michael, 74
Gell-Mann, Murray, 210
gene therapy, promise of, 189
genetic engineering, 202–205, 206
genetics. *See* inheritance
glial cells, described, 21–22
glutamate, transmitter chemicals, 100
glycine, transmitter chemicals, 100
Gould, Elizabeth, 69–70
G protein molecule, neurons, 102
graded potentials:
  electric signals of, 49, 50
  synapse and, 58, 59
gray matter, described, 20, 21
Greenough, William, 144
Gross, Charles, 69–70
growth cone, neurons, 115–116
Guthrie, Arlo, 204
Guthrie, Marjorie, 204
Guthrie, Woody, 204

hallucination, sensory deprivation, 134
Harlow, Harry, 137
Harlow, John, 28–29
hearing:
  brain development, 130
  brain patterns, 135–136
  evolution of, 56
Hebb, Donald O., 160–161, 165, 166–167, 169,
    170, 171, 176, 184
Hebbian synapse, 167
heredity, environment and, 136–137. *See also*
    inheritance
hierarchy, brain structure as, 155
hippocampus:
  aging and, 143–144
  functions of, 40, 41
  memory, 111–114, 134, 175
Hippocrates, 16
Hodgkin, Alan, 42, 44, 46
Hoffman, Klaus, 122
Homo erectus, 12
Homo habilis, 12, 37
Homo sapiens, 12, 13
Hopfield, John, 167
hormones:
  biological clock, 122–123, 125
  brain function and, 57
  mental disorders, 192
  stress, tactile stimulation, 141–142
Hubble, Edwin, 83
Hubel, David, 5, 91, 126, 129, 130, 131, 133,
    136, 137, 138, 148, 171, 209
human genome project, 203
humankind:
  appearance of, 10

  evolution of, 12–13
hunger, sensation and, 56–57
Huntington's disease, 164, 204–205
Huxley, Aldous, 45
Huxley, Andrew, 42, 44, 45–46
hydraulics, 25–26
hydrophobic/hydrophilic amino acids, 104–105
hyperpolarization, 49
hypothalamus, described, 19

illusion, brain function, 72–73
imagination, neuronal ensembles, 172
imipramine, 195–196
immune defense, brain function and, 57
individual differences. *See also* personality;
    subjective experience
  biological clock, 124
  perspective on, 208–209
  sources of, 120
infancy:
  brain development, 141, 144–145, 149, 171
  brain patterns, 136
  language development, 139–140
  nurturing and, 146–147
  reflexes, neuronal ensembles, 178
  tactile stimulation, 141–142
  thalamus, 138
  vision in, 134–135
  visual cortex, 138–139
inheritance. *See also* DNA
  environment and, 136–137
  memory receptors, 175–176
  pharmacology, 200–201
  schizophrenia, 145–146
  subjective experience and, 145
  vision, 135
intelligence, childhood, 144
ion, cell potentials, 43
ion channels:
  function of, 43–44
  molecular action, 105, 106
  neuron, 47
  selectivity of, 48–49
iproniazid, 195

Kant, Immanuel, 95
Katz, Bernard, 91
Kennedy, John F., 7, 13, 211
kinase, molecular action, 113–114
Kline, Nathan, 195
Koch, Christof, 161–162, 163
Kramer, Gustav, 122
Kravitz, Ed, 91, 120
Kuffler, Stephen, 5, 90–92, 97, 98, 129, 130,
    181, 209

Laborit, Henri, 193
La Mettrie, Julien Offroy de, 13, 26
Land, Edwin, 157–158, 159
language. *See also* speech
  age level and, 143
  brain development, 130, 139–140

brain patterns, 135–136
computer and, 168–169
evolution and, 56
importance of, 11
lateral geniculate nucleus (LGN):
  function of, 125
  subjective experience and, 138
lateralization. *See* brain lateralization
L-dopa, 194, 197–198
Leary, Timothy, 199
Leon, Michael, 141
Levi-Montalcini, Rita, 191–192
Libet, Benjamin, 66, 71
light. *See also* photon
  art and, 80
  biological clock, 122, 124–125
  color and, 158, 159–160
  perception of, 83–88
  photon, 76–77
  physics and, 77–78
  relativity theory, 78–80, 209
Linnaeus, Carolus, 121
Linnoila, Markku, 200–201
lithium carbonate, 192–193
Llinás, Rudolfo, 163, 164, 165, 179, 181–182, 183–184, 185, 209
Locke, John, 136
locked-in state, biofeedback, 63
long-term potentiation (LTP), 113–114, 175

magnesium ions, cell potentials, 43
magnetic resonance imaging (MRI), 15–16, 17
mapping. *See* brain mapping
mathematical calculations:
  array of sensory vectors, 182–183, 184
  neurons, 180–181
matrix, array of sensory vectors, 182–183, 184
Maxwell, James, 77
meditation, 163
medulla oblongata, described, 18–19
memory:
  Alzheimer's disease, 116–118
  brain and, 40
  brain cell generation, 70
  hippocampus, 111–114, 134
  molecular action, 111
  neuronal ensembles, 174–176
  vision and, 134–135
Mendel, Gregor Johann, 137
mental disorders:
  hormones, 192
  neuronal ensembles, 178–179
  pharmacology, 192–202, 206
Michelangelo, 24
microscope, brain research and, 5
midbrain, visual neural pathways, 154
mind/body relationship:
  brain and, 73
  current science, 208
  historical perspective on, 26
molecular action:
  Alzheimer's disease, 116–118

memory, 111
neurons, 102–103
photon and, 102, 109–111
protein molecules, 103–109
monoamines, 194, 195, 196
Morton, William, 51
mothering, importance of, 137
motion:
  action and, 101
  cerebellum, 181, 185
  neuronal calculations, 180–181
  vision and, 149–153
Müller, Johannes, 51, 57
Mullins, Kary, 203
multiple sclerosis, 21
myelin, 20, 21
myosin, growth cone, 116

National Aeronautics and Space Administration (NASA), 14–15
nerve growth factor (NGF), 191–192
NETtalk computer, 168–169
neural network computer, 167–169
neurobiology, development of, 91, 129
neuroimaging, development of, 15–16
neuromodulators, 60, 107, 109
neuronal ensembles (cell assemblies), 170–179
  cognition, 177
  formation of, 170–172
  memory, 174–176
  mental disorders, 178–179
  perception, 172–174
  reflexes, 178
neurons:
  autoradiology, 120–121
  binding problem, 161
  brain adaptation, 137–138
  brain function, 7–8, 20–23, 30–31, 39, 40
  cerebellum, 181–182
  communication between, 14
  cortical, visual cortex, 130–131
  DNA and, 48
  electric signals of, 49–50
  emotion, 185–186
  evolution of, 46
  firing of, 162–163, 166–167, 169–170
  gated ion channels, 47
  generation of, in brain, 69–70
  growth cone, 115–116
  mathematical calculations by, 180–181
  mental activity, 186–187
  molecular action in, 102–103
neuronal ensembles (cell assemblies), 170–179 (*See also* neuronal ensembles (cell assemblies))
  personality, 187, 208–209
  reaction time and, 11
  receptive fields of, 96–97
  recording of signals of, 63–65, 161
  stroke patients, 142–143
  subjective experience and, 68–69

neuronal ensembles (*continued*)
  synapse and, 58–60
  taste and, 10
neuropharmacology. *See* pharmacology
neuroscience:
  defined, 9
  growth of, 14–15, 99
neurotransmitters, pharmacology, 198
Newton, Isaac, 77, 78, 79, 80, 158
Nicholson, Jack, 179
N-methyl D-aspartate (NMDA) receptor:
  aging, 143–144
  memory, 111–114
nonchannel linked receptors, molecular
    action, 106–109
nondominant hemisphere, 36
norepinephrine, 189, 194, 195, 199, 200

obsessive-compulsive disorder, neuronal
    ensembles, 178–179
occipital lobe:
  color vision, 159
  visual cortex and, 132
  visual neural pathways, 154
olfaction:
  chemical receptors, 54, 55
  survival and, 11–12
ophthalmology, perception and, 51–52
optic nerves, biological clock, 122
Ortous de Mairain, Jean Jacques d', 121

pain, perception of, 55
parasympathetic nervous system, described,
    190
parietal lobe, visual neural pathways,
    153–155
Parkinson's disease, 40, 109, 163–164, 194,
    197
patterns, brain and, 133–136
Paxil, 197
Pellionisz, Andras, 183, 185
Penfield, Wilder, 32, 42, 67, 69
Penrose, Roger, 74
perception. *See also* sensation
  behavior and, 182
  binding problem, 160–161
  evolution and, 54–56
  light, 83–88
  neuronal ensembles, 172–174
  physics of, 52–53
  sensation and, 51–52, 56–57
  subjective experience and, 52–53
  visual cortex and, 136
Perkel, D. H., 183, 185
personality. *See also* subjective experience;
    individual differences
  brain injury and, 28–29
  neurons, 187, 208–209
  perception and, 182
Petty, Peter G., 208
pharmacology:
  Alzheimer's disease, 118

current status, 205–206
historical perspective, 190–205
neuromodulators, 109
research in, 188–189
stroke patient rehabilitation, 142–143
pheromones, chemical receptors, 54–55
philosophy:
  perception and sensation, 51–52
  science and, 3, 210–211
photon. *See also* light
  evolution and, 81, 83
  molecular action and, 102, 109–111
  production of, 76–77
  speed of light and, 88
  vision and, 76, 98–99
photoreceptors:
  activation of, 98–99
  development of, 81–83
  ganglion cells, 91–98
  light perception, 85–88, 89–90
photosynthesis, 84
phrenology, 27–28
physics:
  light and, 77–78
  Newtonian, 77
  vision, 52–53
pineal gland, biological clock, 122
pituitary gland:
  biological clock, 122, 125
  described, 19
plants, timekeeping by, 121
Plato, 3
poisons, protection from, 57
polymerase chain reaction (PCR), 202,
    203–204
pons, described, 18–19
positron emission tomography (PET):
  brain mapping, 25, 171, 172
  development of, 16
  obsessive-compulsive disorder, 179
postsynaptic membrane, 58
potassium ions:
  cell potentials, 43
  ion channels, 44
prefrontal cortex, subjective experience and,
    69
presynaptic membrane, 58
proprioceptors, function of, 55
protein molecules, molecular action, 103–109
proteomics, 118
Prozac, 197, 198
psychotherapy, neuronal ensembles, 178

qualia, subjective experience, 67, 68, 208
quarks, 210
Quartz, Steven, 70

Ramey, Craig, 144
Ramón y Cajal, Santiago, 13–14, 115, 181, 211
rapid-eye-movement sleep, electroencephalog-
    raphy, 61–62
Rauwolfia serpentina, 194–195

INDEX

reaction time:
  brain, 41
  neurons and, 11
readiness potential, free will, 71
receptive fields:
  ganglion cells, 91–98
  neurons, 96–97
receptor enzyme molecule, neurons, 102
recombinant DNA, 202–203
recording techniques, neuronal signals,
  63–65
Reeve, Christopher, 206
reflexes:
  neuronal ensembles, 178, 187
  superior colliculi, 127–128
rehabilitation, stroke patients, 142–143
Reisch, Gregor, 23–25, 171–172
relativity theory, 78–80, 209
religion:
  mind/body relationship, 26, 27
  spirit and, 13
Renaissance, 24–25
repetition, neuronal ensembles, 178
research. See also pharmacology
  advances in, 2–4
  historical perspective on, 5, 13–20
  limits of, 4
  space exploration and, 57
reserpine, 195, 196
respiration, sensation and, 56
resting membrane potential, 43, 44–45
restriction enzymes, 202–203
restrictive fragment length polymorphisms
  (RFLPs), 205
retina. See also eye; vision
  biological clock, 121, 124–125
  brain and, 81–83
  fetal development, 125–127
  ganglion cells, 91–98
  lateral geniculate nucleus (LGN), 125
  light perception, 87–88
  visual cortex and, 132
rods, light perception, 85–86
Rosenberg, Charles, 168

saccades, 151
Sacks, Oliver, 72
schizophrenia, 109
  inheritance and subjective experience,
    145–146
  pharmacology, 195
Schoenbaum, Geoffrey, 170
science, philosophy and, 3, 210–211
scopolamine, 191
Searle, John, 66
Sejnowski, Terry, 168
sensation. See also perception
  neuronal ensembles, 172
  perception and, 51–52, 56–57
sensory deprivation, brain patterns and,
  133–134, 163
sensory receptor, transducer and, 57–58

sensory stimulation, brain development, 139,
  141–142
serotonin, 60, 194, 195, 199–201
serotonin reuptake inhibitors (SSRIs), 197
Seurat, George, 87
severe combined immune deficiency (SCID),
  189
Shatz, Carla, 127
Simon, Jennifer Jones, 204
Simon, Norton, 204
skin, tactile receptors, 55
skull, 22
sleep, electroencephalography, 61–62
smell. See olfaction
smile, origins of, 22, 23
Snyder, Solomon, 198
social implications, pharmacology, 201–202
sodium ions:
  cell potentials, 43
  ion channels, 44, 48–49
  transmitter chemicals, 100
sodium-potassium pump, function of, 44, 45
space exploration, 2
  medical applications of, 14–15
  research advances and, 57
space/time continuum:
  biological clock, 123–124
  relativity theory, 78–80, 209
species-specific functions:
  biological clock, 123
  brain, 53–54
speech. See also language
  brain mapping and, 29–30
  evolution and, 56
spirit:
  brain function and, 16–18, 25
  religion and, 13
stem cells, 206
stress hormones, tactile stimulation, 141–142
Stretton, Tony, 120
stroke patients, rehabilitation of, 142–143,
  171
subjective experience. See also personality;
    individual differences
  behavior and, 137
  brain cell generation, 70
  brain function and, 4, 8–10, 80
  brain mapping and, 67–69
  brain neurons and, 137–138
  brain patterns, 136
  glial cells, 21–22
  inheritance and, 145
  neuronal firing, 166, 187
  neuronal recordings and, 65
  perception and, 52–53
  perspective on, 208–209
  qualia, 67
  schizophrenia, 145–146
  vision and, 83
substantia nigra, Parkinson's disease, 40
suicide, pharmacology, 199–200, 201
superior colliculi, visual maps, 127–128

INDEX

supra-chiasmatic nucleus (SCN), biological
  clock, 122–123
survival:
  fitness and, 11–12
species-specific brain function, 53–54
sympathetic nervous system, described,
  189–190
synapses:
  neuronal ensembles, 178
  neuronal firing and, 166–167, 169–170
  neurons and, 58–60
  transmitter chemicals, 99–100
synaptic cleft, 58
synaptic plasticity, 171

tactile receptors, skin, 55
tactile stimulation, infancy, 141–142
Tai chi, 184, 185
taste:
  neurons and, 10
  perception of, 183
temperature, perception of, 55
temporal lobe, visual neural pathways to, 153
thalamo-cortical signals, brain disease,
  164–165
thalamus:
  attention, 162–163
  fetal development, 126
  functions of, 40, 41, 125, 162–163
  Parkinson's disease, 163–164
  subjective experience and, 138
theory of relativity, 78–80, 209
theta waves, electroencephalography, 61
thirst, sensation and, 56–57
Thorazine, 193–194, 195, 196, 198
time. See reaction time
time keeping. See biological clock
time/space continuum. See space/time
  continuum
Tinbergen, Nickolaas, 135
Tomita, Tsuneo, 98
touch, perception of, 55
toxins, protection from, 57
transducer, sensory receptor and, 57–58
transmitter chemicals, synapse, 99–100
transmitter molecule:
  chemically-gated ion channels, 47
  molecular action, 105
tricyclic antidepressants, 196
tryptophan, 200
Tsien, Joe Z., 112–113, 114, 143
Twin studies, schizophrenia, 146

uncertainty principle, 74

ventricles:
  brain cell generation, 70, 206

cerebrospinal fluid, 22
  historical research on, 16–18, 25
vestibular apparatus, evolution of, 55–56
vestibular reflex, motion and, 150
Vinci, Leonardo da, 24, 87
violence:
  child neglect and, 146–147
  pharmacology, 199–201
viruses, chemical receptors, 55
vision. See also eye; retina
  brain adaptation, 137–138
  brain function, 81
  brain injury, 30, 151–152
  evolution of, 56
  ganglion cells, 89–90, 91–98
  infancy, 134–135
  motion and, 149–153
  photon and, 76
  physics of, 52–53
  process of, 84–85
  subjective experience and, 83
  survival and, 11
visual cortex injury, 156–157
visual cortex:
  blindness and, 132–133
  cortical neurons and, 130–131
  fetal development, 125–126
  function of, 131–132
  infancy, 138–139
  injury, 153–154, 156
  pathways from, 148–149
  study of, 129
visual flow, 152
visual maps, superior colliculi, 127–128
visual pigment, 83–88, 111
vitamin A, 86, 111
voltage-gated ion channels:
  function of, 47
  molecular action, 106
  selectivity of, 48–49

Wald, George, 83, 86, 97, 102, 109, 111
Watson, James, 161, 202
Wernicke, Carl, 30
Wernicke's area, language development, 140
Wexler, Alice, 204
Wexler, Milton, 204
Wexler, Nancy, 204
white blood cells, brain function and, 57
white matter, described, 20
Wiesel, Torsten, 5, 91, 129, 130, 131, 133, 136,
  137, 138, 148, 171, 209

Yamamoto, Keith, 118

Zeki, Semir, 155–156, 159
Zoloft, 197